GIMME MY
SSA DISABILITY!

*The step-by-step disability
guide to help you get the disability benefits you deserve*

Beth Losure

Table of Contents

GIMME MY SSA DISABILITY!

2.5 million disability applications were file last year. Out of the millions of applications submitted, however, the Social Security Administration (SSA) approved a paltry 32%.

What does that mean for you? If you are desperate and disabled you need SSDI now, before you have to wait months (and yes, possibly years) to get benefits.

Trolling the internet will help you understand some of what you need to know, but who has the time to devote hours to mindless and often fruitless online searches, or worse yet, to read a three hundred page disability book!

The good news is many applicants are only denied SSDI benefits because they do not understand a few simple concepts– how to verify their work credits, how to prove they are disabled, or what type of medical information they need to provide to prove their case. Each of these roadblocks, however, can be overcome with a little bit of time and research.

Although there are some great books that you can read, most of them do not provide a simple plan. That's all changed with GIMME MY SSA DISABILITY! This guide provides detailed, step-by-step instructions. It tells you exactly what you need to do at every step of the disability process. It is a simple guide with hard-hitting truths about what you need to know to get SSDI benefits the first time you apply.

Who can benefit from this guide?

- Those with a severe health condition

- Those whose condition will last at least 12 continuous months

- Those who cannot work

This guide is not intended for those who do not want to get a job, those who think getting disability benefits is easier than getting a job (it isn't), or those who want to play golf while the rest of America works.

If you can work, you need to work. Too many workers apply for benefits when they do not qualify. This backs up the application process for millions of other Americans who desperately need SSDI benefits.

Before applying for SSDI, verify you meet the SSDI requirements by reading this guide.

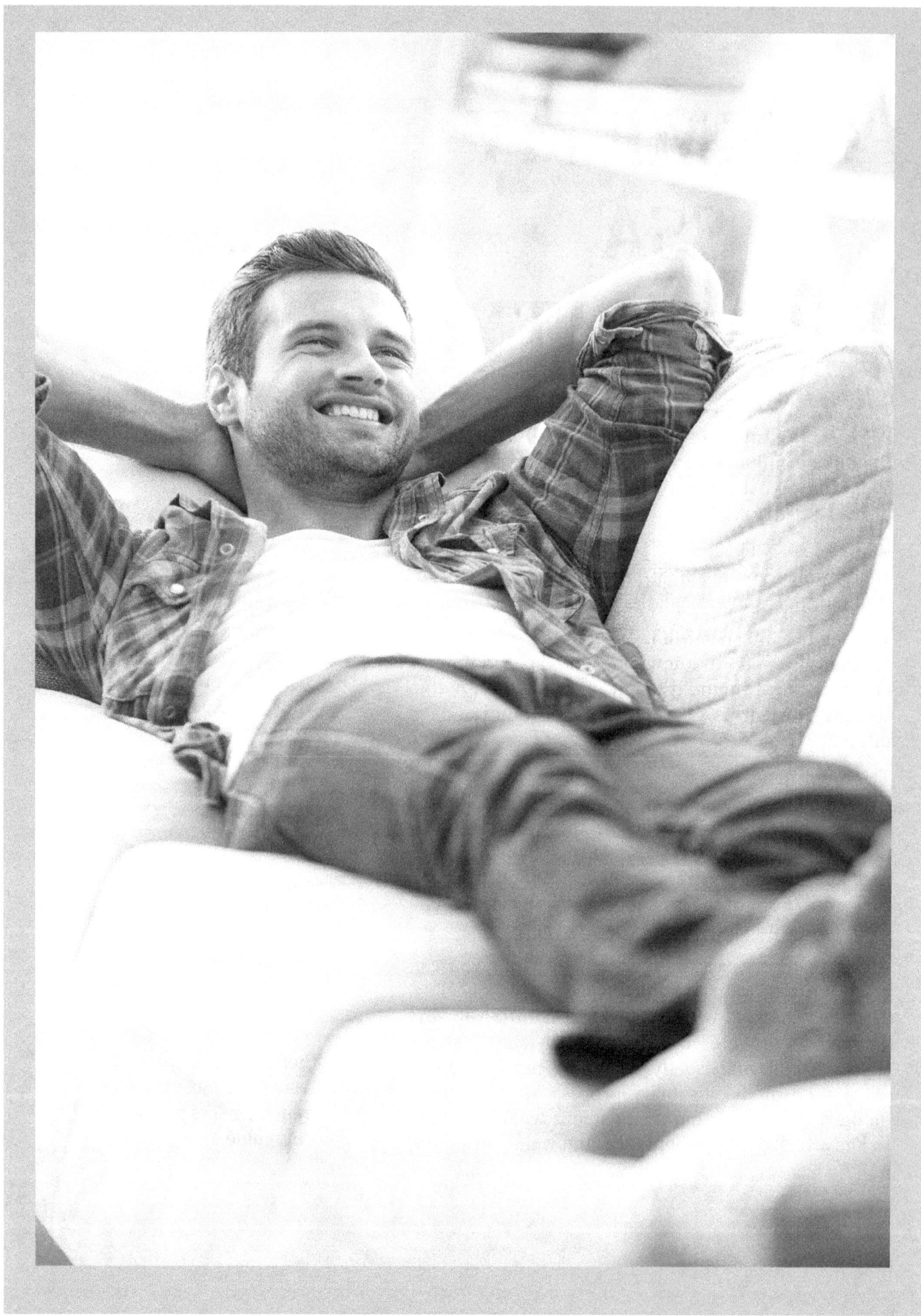

Getting in the right frame of mind...

If you are applying for SSDI benefits it's time to take a deep breath and prepare yourself for what's ahead. Applying and qualifying for SSDI is not something that will happen in one day or one week. Although some claimants are approved or fast-tracked for benefits, most are not. For most claimants, getting SSDI disability benefits is a very long process. More importantly, it's imperative to understand that most claimants are denied the first time they apply for SSDI benefits.

The good news is there are more resources and more help available to claimants than ever before. Not only are there thousands of articles online, there are also dozens of books, disability advocates, and disability lawyers all willing to provide applicants with help.

Historically, claimants had to rely on the Social Security Administration for help. Not anymore. With a little time and effort, you can get the right information to improve your chances of winning benefits. What you will need to do, however, is to take it slowly and review all the information you need to win benefits BEFORE you apply.

The best type of SSDI applicant is a well-informed applicant. Ignore advice, refuse to do your research, and apply before you understand the process and you will have difficulty getting approved for Social Security Disability Insurance (SSDI).

Review this Guide and follow every step in the process. If you still have questions after you have read this Guide, you can email me at beth.losure@yahoo.com and I will be glad to help you.

Are you ready to begin? Let's review the first thing you need to know before applying for Social Security Disability Insurance (SSDI).

STEP: 1

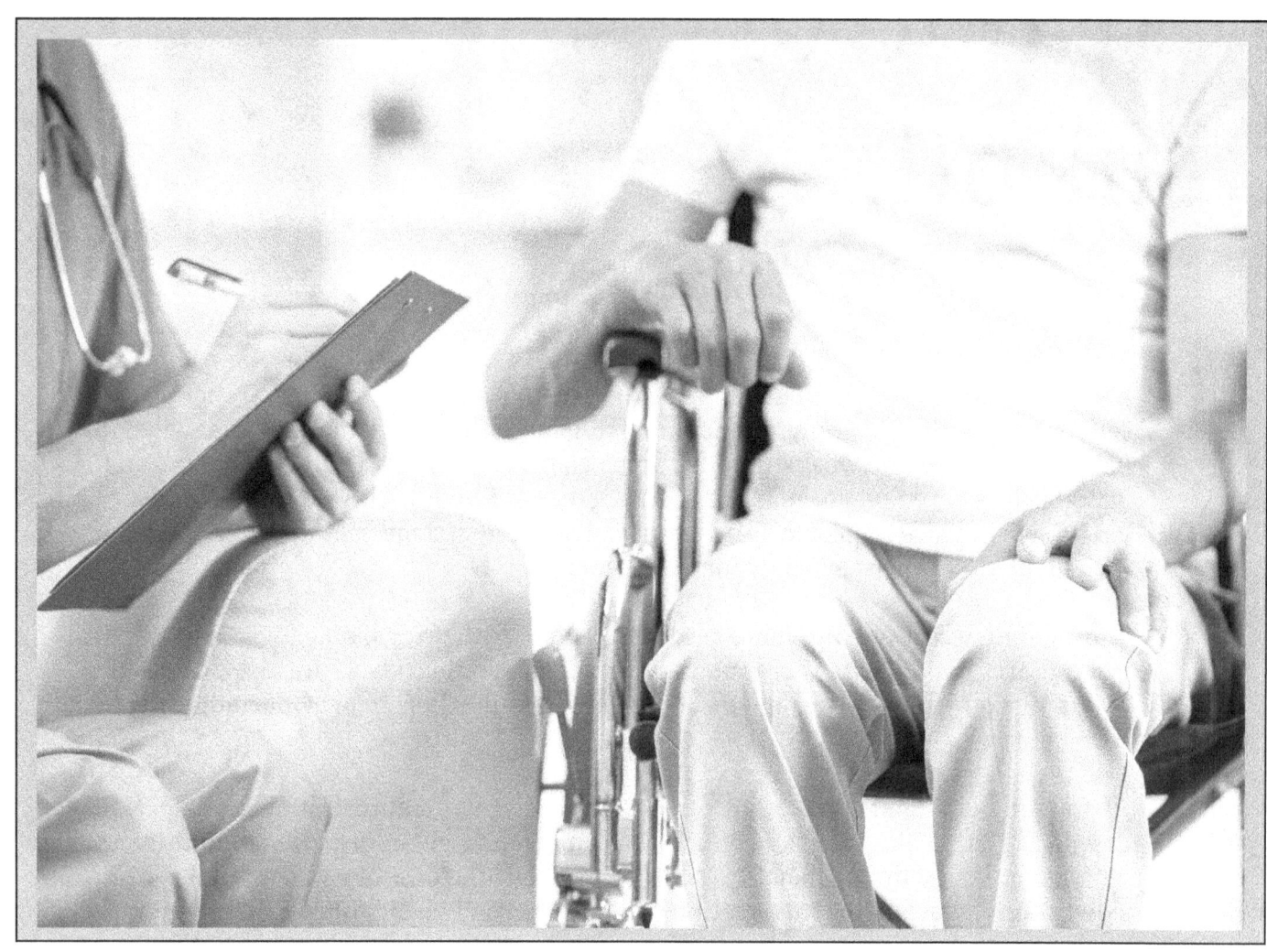

Do I understand SSDI?

Do I understand SSDI?

Social Security Disability Insurance (SSDI) is a wage replacement program for disabled workers who meet certain non-medical and medical requirements. SSDI auxiliary benefits may also be paid to the children and spouses of certain disabled workers.

No, you are not *entitled* to SSDI benefits, and you will not be awarded benefits just because you have worked thirty years laying asphalt in the hot, Texas sun.

SSDI is not like SSA retirement benefits. You will not get SSDI just because you filled out an application and sent it to the Social Security Administration. In fact, unless you do your research, you will probably be denied SSDI the first time you apply.

Why you will probably be denied SSDI...

Yes, there are some claimants who spend hours researching how to qualify for benefits, gathering their medical records (which you do not need to do), and talking to friends and family. They sit down ready to fill out their application with every bit of information they need.

But let's be honest, that's probably not you. In fact, you probably have no idea where to start, whether you need to call the SSA, or whether you can complete an application online.

You're uninformed, which is understandable given the thousands of pages of regulations that only a seasoned disability lawyer can truly understand. You do, however, need to be realistic about your chances of getting SSDI benefits the first time you apply, especially if you do not understand the basics of how the SSA makes a disability decision.

Supplemental Security Income > Do not get confused

The Social Security Administration (SSA) has two separate programs which offer disability benefits: Social Security Disability Insurance (SSDI) and Supplemental Security Income (SSI). This book specifically deals with the Social Security Disability Insurance or SSDI program.

Supplemental Security Income (SSI) is offered to the aged, the blind, and the disabled who are unable to work for at least 12 continuous months. SSI recipients must also have very limited income and resources. SSI recipients do not, however, have to work or have work credits to qualify for SSI benefits. SSI applicants can, however, be disqualified if they are married to a spouse who makes too much money or they are receiving assistance from others.

STEP: 2

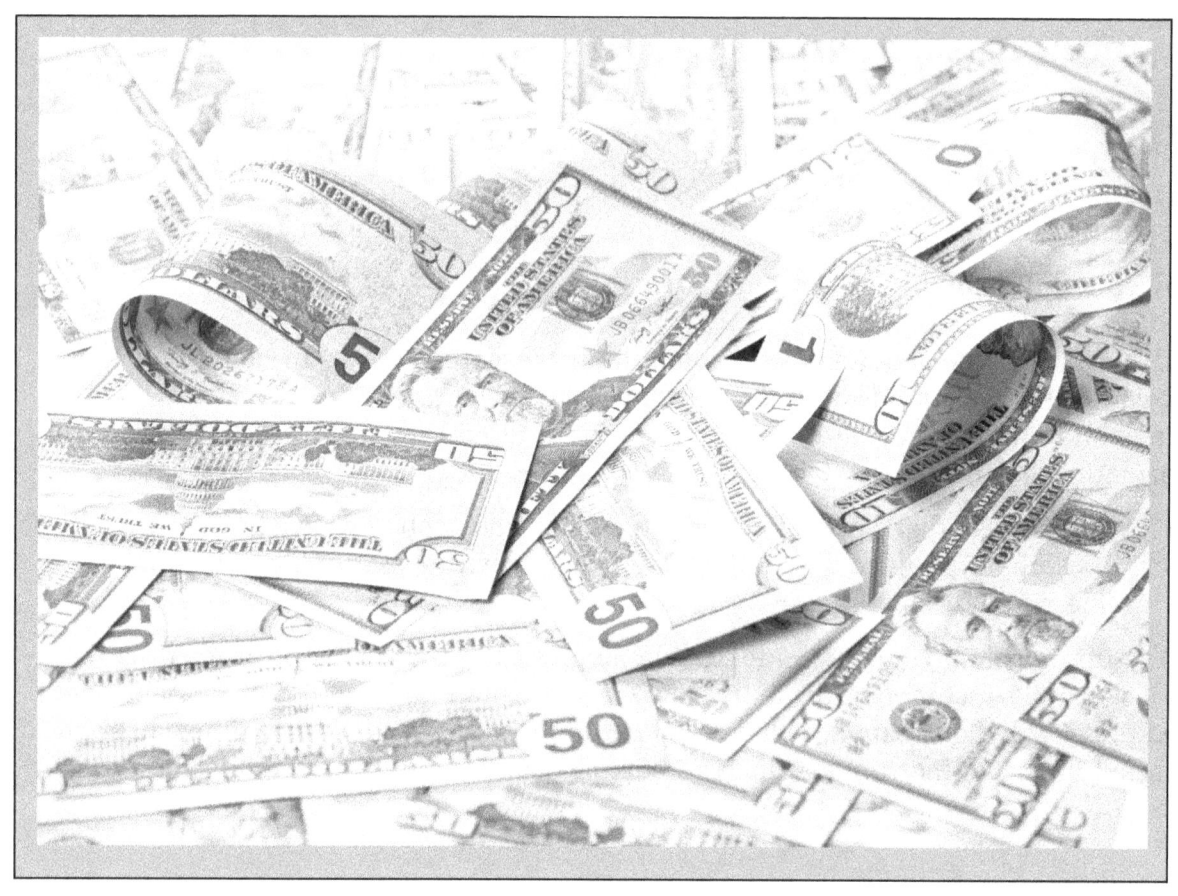

Do I meet the nonmedical requirements for SSDI?

Do I meet the non-medical requirements for SSDI?

Non-medical requirements for SSDI generally include financial and legal requirements -- issues that have nothing to do with your medical conditions or medical eligibility. If you do not meet these requirements the SSA does not care how sick you are...I'm serious, they do not care. You will be denied SSDI benefits.

1. Review your work credits

Workers must work, pay taxes, and earn work credits to be ensured for SSDI. And no, working and getting paid "under the table" by your Uncle Fred will not get it done. f you have not worked and have not paid sufficient taxes, you are not insured, and you will not qualify for SSDI benefits, regardless of the severity of your health condition.

Work credits cannot be bought or borrowed, which means you cannot go and ask your wife or cousin Ed if you can borrow a few of their credits.

If you do not have enough work credits contact the SSA and see if you can qualify for Supplemental Security Income (SSI). You can also attempt to go back to work, which, unfortunately, is probably not an option or you would not be applying for SSDI.

IMPORTANT!!

The number of work credits you will need to qualify for SSDI benefits will depend on your age when you became disabled. Most people will need 40 work credits, 20 of which must be earned in the 10 years ending with the year they became disabled (exceptions for the blind exist).

The amount needed to earn one work credit also changes. For example, in 2016, claimants could earn one credit for every $1,260 of wages or self-employment income. Claimants can earn up to 4 credits a year. Review www.ssa.gov for more information about the amount of wages it takes each year to generate a work credit.

Workers who have not worked enough and earned enough in wages to generate work credits will not qualify for SSDI benefits. Claimants without work credits may talk to the SSA about whether or not they might qualify for Supplemental Security Income (SSI).

How to find your work credits...

There are three ways to find out if you have enough work credits for SSDI benefits:

1. Go online

Visiting the SSA website at www.ssa.gov/myaccount is by far the easiest way to find out if you qualify for SSDI benefits. After you sign in you can do the following:

- Verify and track your earnings
- Get an estimate of your future benefits
- Manage your benefits

2. Call the SSA at 1-800-772-1213

If you do decide to call the SSA you could be on hold for a significant amount of time. Prepare yourself for the wait.

3. Look at your paper statement

Although the SSA used to send out a statement every year, this was stopped. Now the SSA will only send them out every five years for those aged 25 to 60 who are not registered online. Review your statement to determine what benefits you and your family may be eligible to receive under certain conditions.

Disability benefit information is located on the second page of your SSA Statement. If you qualify for SSDI you should see a statement which says something like this:

Disability You have earned enough credits to qualify for benefits. If you became disabled right now, your payment would be about...$ 1,527/month

Your benefit payment estimate will vary from the listed amount here and is based on your average earnings and the amount of taxes you have paid. To estimate your benefits you can also use the SSA benefits calculator located on the SSA site at www.ssa.gov

IMPORTANT!!!! WORK CREDITS EXPIRE

Work credits expire!! There is a date in the future called your Date Last Insured (DLI). If you stop working and wait too long to apply there will be a point in time in which you no longer qualify for SSDI. It will not matter that you worked thirty years. If you wait too long to apply, you could lose your eligibility for SSDI.

Do not stop working and wait years to apply for SSDI. If you are disabled and cannot work it's important to apply for benefits right away. If you cannot immediately complete your application contact the SSA and ask about establishing your protective filing date.

2. Make sure you are under your full retirement age

Workers who have reached the full retirement age will not qualify for SSDI benefits. Instead, they will need to apply for SSA retirement.

If you are receiving SSDI benefits when you reach your full retirement age your benefits are converted to SSA retirement. You will not receive both retirement and SSDI.. I know, that's a bummer!

If you are close to your full retirement age you need to talk to the SSA to determine if it's better to take early retirement or file for disability.

Your early retirement payment could be less than your disability benefit, but it may be harder to qualify for SSDI.

3. Make sure you meet the residency requirements

SSDI is generally only available to U.S. citizens. Of course, there are exceptions, and if you are interested (and you need a nap) you can google 8 U.S.C. 1612 Limited Eligibility of Qualified Aliens for Certain Federal Programs.

If you doo not meet the age or residency requirements for Social Security Disability Insurance (SSDI), your SSDI application will be denied before the SSA review your medical condition.

NOTE:

All of your non- medical requirements are reviewed at your local Social Security Administration Office.

If you do not have enough work credits, you are too old, or you do not meet the residency requirements, the SSA will automatically deny your SSDI application.

Work credit denials, which are referred to as technical denials, can be challenged if you have evidence the SSA made the calculation incorrectly. If this is the case, you will need to contact the SSA within 60 days from the receipt of your denial and talk to them about how to appeal your denial.

You may also be able to file for Supplemental Security Income (SSI) if you do not have enough work credits for SSDI. Generally, the SSA will determine if you are eligible for SSI at the time you are denied for SSDI, which means you may not have to submit another application. Talk to the SSA if you have questions.

Non-medical requirements (cont.)

4. Determine if you working too much or making too much money

The SSA has this fancy term for work: substantial gainful activity. What this really means is that if you are working too many hours or making too much money, you are not disabled.

The SSA will not care that you have a severe health condition but you get up and struggle through work each day. If you work too much or make too much money, the SSA will consider you NOT disabled.

What is gainful work?

In 2016, gainful work is making $1,130 per month (for the non-blind). This amount is updated periodically by the SSA. Work can also be gainful, however, if it is normally done for pay or profit, even if it is not generating a profit, and work that is intended for pay or profit, even if profit is not realized.

Bottom line: if you are working at a job that generally generates profit you can still be denied SSDI, even if you are not currently earning a profit (i.e., trying to start a small business but you are not making money).

What is substantial work?

The amount of work the SSA considers substantial is a bit unclear. Forty hours is definitely substantial, but let's assume you work thirty-five. In some cases, the SSA may decide you could work a bit more and consider you not disabled.

This is true even if the work does not generate gainful activity. For example, if you performed 40 hours of volunteer work each week the SSA would consider you not disabled even though you are not making a profit. The SSA's assumption is that if you can do 40 hours of volunteer work, you also have the capability to work 40 hours for pay.

BOTTOM LINE:

YOU WILL NOT BE AWARDED SSDI BENEFITS IF YOU ARE WORKING TOO MANY HOURS OR/AND MAKING TOO MUCH MONEY, DESPITE THE SEVERITY OF YOUR HEALTH CONDITION.

What are my options if I do not have enough work credits?

Unfortunately, if you do not have enough work credits for SSDI, and you decided to apply anyway, you will be denied benefits.

Although some type of denials can be appealed, the only chance you would have to overturn this denial decision is to prove that the SSA made a miscalculation or that they did not have all of your employment data. This is referred to as a technical denial.

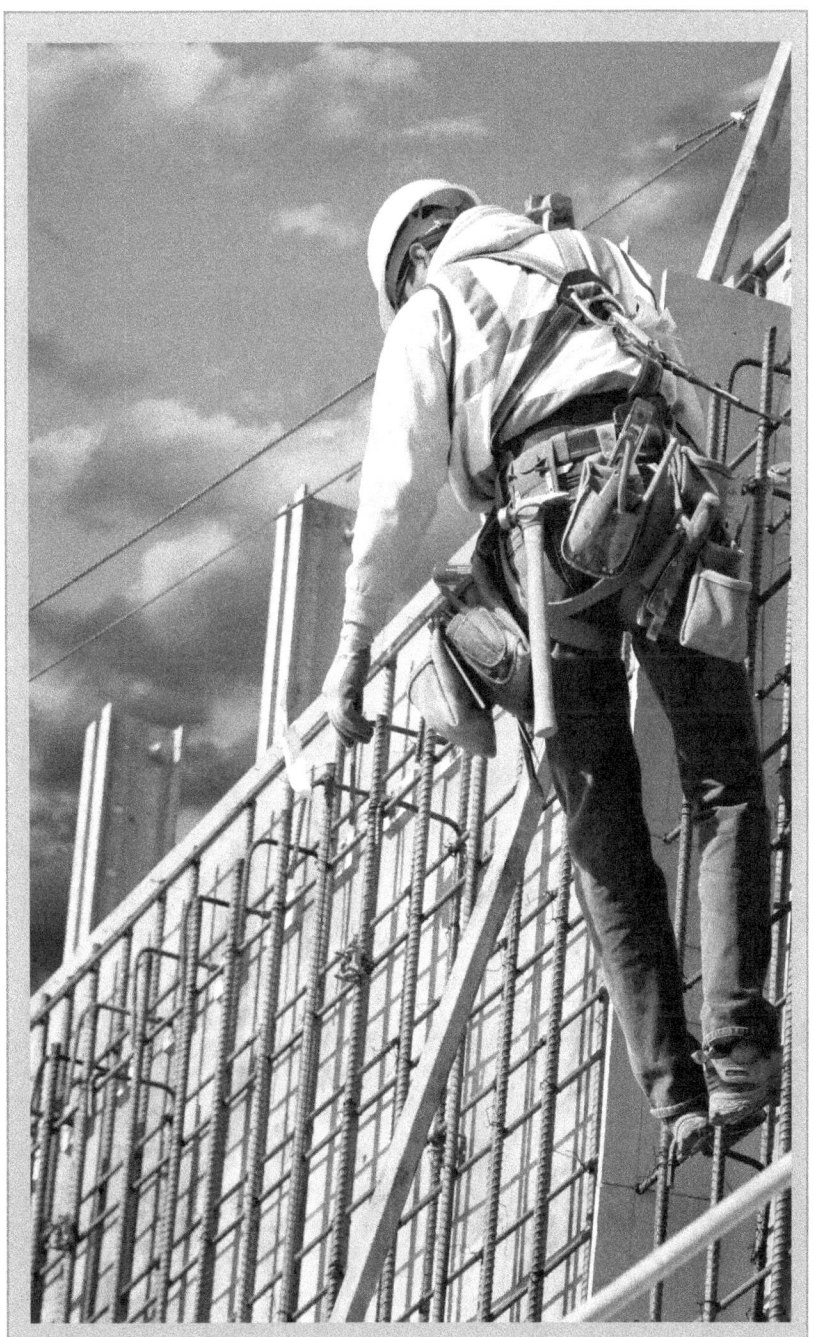

Option after a SSDI denial for insufficient work credits:

1. **Go back to work**

Some claimants may have been denied because they did not have enough work credits. If you are shy only a few work credits returning to work and working very part-time for a few months may help you earn enough work credits to qualify for SSDI benefits.

2. **Apply for SSI**

Some SSDI applicants may qualify for SSI benefits if they do not have enough work credits for SSDI and they have very limited income and resources.

3. **Do nothing**

Although this is not an option for all claimants, some claimants who are married or have other means of supporting themselves may simply stop working and do nothing.

STEP: 3

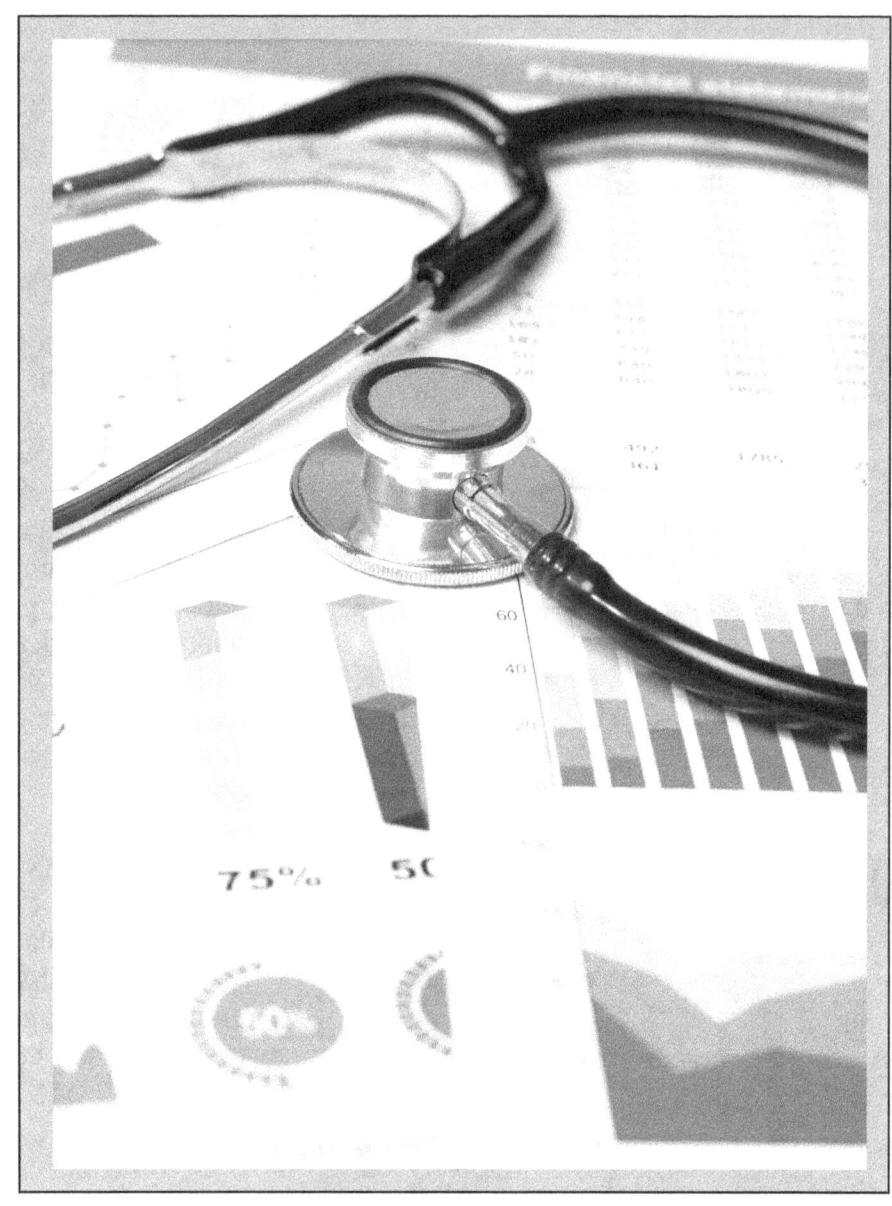

Do I meet the medical requirements for SSDI?

Do I meet the medical requirements for SSDI?

To understand the medical requirements for SSDI benefits you need to know what the SSA considers disabled. They defined disabled as the following:

"The inability to engage in any substantial gainful activity by reason of any medically physical or mental impairment which can be expected to result in death or which will last no less than 12 continuous months."

To quote Tom Cruise, "I don't know what they means, but it sounds bad." Just kidding,. Let's break it down so you know exactly what that means. The question we are really getting at is whether or not you are disabled, which we will discuss in more detail later in the book.

At this step, however, let's just look at the basic questions you need to answer to decide if you meet the medical requirements to qualify for SSDI and whether or not you should pursue a claim.

Question 1: Are you currently working or can you work?

We discussed substantial gainful activity in the last section. As mentioned, if you are working and making too much money your claim will be denied by the SSA local office. IF YOU ARE WORKING NOW AND MAKING TOO MUCH MONEY, DO NOT BOTHER APPLYING. YOUR CASE WILL BE DENIED.

Sorry to keep shouting, but thousands of claimants apply every year despite working full-time, and it mucks the process up for everyone else.

Now to the second part of the question. What if you apply and you are not currently working? If you absolutely cannot work, keep reading. If you have not been able to find a job but you could work, or you simply do not want to work– close this guide and hit the pavement.

What if you cannot work for at least a year so you apply for benefits but then go back to work after 12 months? You may qualify for closed period benefits, which means you can be paid for the 12 months you were out of work (less the five month waiting period to get SSDI).

Over 2 million people apply for SSDI and SSI benefits each year. Over two million people are NOT 100% disabled. Do not apply if you are not disabled. It wastes the time and resources of those who are truly disabled. If you are not disabled but you cannot work your current job it may be time to find a job you can work. Can you retrain or go back to school? Is there a sedentary job that you can perform? Can you work part-time? If you are not 100% disabled you need to find something you can do.

Do I meet the medical requirements (cont.)

Question 2: Do you have a severe health condition?

Get ready, this one is a doozy. According to the SSA, a severe health condition is:

"A medically determinable impairment that results from an anatomical, physiological, or psychological abnormality which can be proven by medically acceptable clinical and laboratory diagnostic techniques."

Let's break that down into real English. Basically, it's saying that you have to have a real mental or physical condition, and you need medical information from your doctor that lists the diagnosis and prognosis. Throw in some clinical tests, laboratory results, and diagnostic testing, and you are good to go!

I'd give you one little bit of advice. Before you apply for SSDI make sure you have gone to the doctor and have a diagnosis. It's tough to convince the SSA you have a severe health condition if no one knows what it is.

Keep in mind, as I mentioned before, it is possible for you to think your condition is severe but you have kept working. You need to decide, however, is it so severe you cannot work? If you can work the SSA will automatically consider your condition not severe, (regardless of whether or not it really is severe).

Warning:
There is also a risk if you start to work part-time for several years. Your SSDI payment is based on your average earnings and the taxes you pay. If your earning substantially decline, your SSDI payment may decline too.

All of your medical requirements are reviewed at the Disability Determinations Services Office for your state. Details about how the DDS makes their disability decision can be found under Step 6 What do I need to understand about the SSDI application process?

Each DDS office is supposed to follow the same processes to make a disability determination for each claimant. If after the DDS requests your medical information they do not have sufficient information to make a disability determination they may ask you to see a consultative examiner, who is an objective medical evaluator who will provide more information about your condition to the DDS so the DDS can make a more informed decision.

Question 3: Will your condition last at least 12 continuous months?

The SSA does not offer any type of short-term disability benefits. The reason they give is that they believe that most people have the resources to plan for short-term, unexpected health issues. Uh...probably not, but regardless, they do not offer any benefits if your condition is not going to last at least 12 continuous months.

Now, here's another kick to the pants. It does not matter how severely you are injured right at this moment. You could be completely paralyzed, laying in a hospital bed and in a coma. If your condition is expected to improve within 12 months, you are not disabled. If your condition will not last 12 continuous months– DO NOT APPLY!

Disability Checklist

Continue reading if all of the following are true:

⇒ I am not working too much or making too much money.
⇒ I have seen a doctor and I have a diagnosis and a prognosis for my condition.
⇒ I meet the SSDI residency requirements.
⇒ I have worked, paid taxes. and verified my work credits.
⇒ I have a condition which will last at least 12 continuous months.
⇒ I have a severe health condition.
⇒ I am less than my full retirement age.
⇒ I medical records to support my claims.

Do not keep reading or apply for SSDI benefits if any of the following are true:

⇒ I have not seen a doctor and I refuse to see one.
⇒ I do not have any medical evidence to support my case.
⇒ I do not have any work credits and I will not qualify for SSI benefits.
⇒ I do not have a severe condition.
⇒ I do not have a condition which will last 12 continuous months.
⇒ I am greater than my full retirement age.

STEP: 4

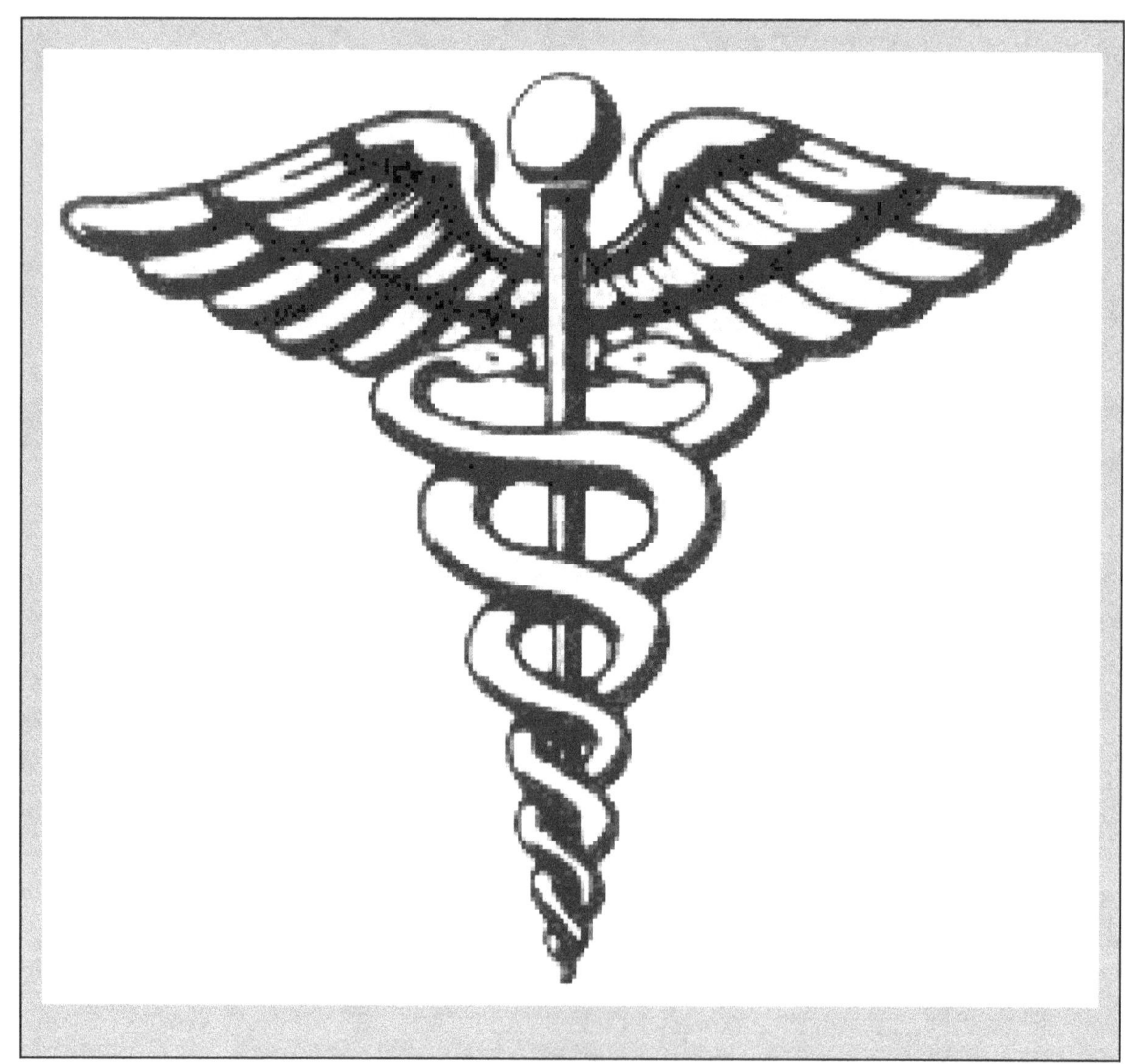

Do I have the medical evidence to prove my SSDI claim?

Do I have the medical evidence to prove my SSDI claim?

Step 1: Verify you have medical evidence to support each disability you list on your application

Make sure you have medical evidence to prove every impairment you list on your disability application. This is probably the hardest and most important thing you need to do to improve your chances of winning SSDI.

The SSA will make their disability determination almost entirely on the evidence provided by you or your doctors to them about your disabling health conditions.

I hate to be Debbie Downer, especially given the sorry state of the healthcare system in the United States, but I think it's safe to say, for most claimants, it will be nearly impossible to win benefits without any medical records.

I will repeat. Avoid applying for SSDI- if at all possible– if you do not have medical evidence to support your case. If you do not have medical evidence the SSA may send you to a consultative examiner for a medical evaluation, but this exam does not help most claimants get approved.

It's always better to have an established relationship with a doctor who understands your condition!!

What do I do if I do not have medical evidence?

Not having medical evidence can severely jeopardize your SSDI claim. With this in mind, if you do not have insurance or a medical doctor you will need to get more creative to get medical care and ensure you have enough information to prove your case. It will not be easy, but here are some steps you can take:

⇒ Rely on the consultative medical examination

⇒ Go to your own doctor and ask if they will take reduced payments

⇒ Go to a minor emergency center regularly

⇒ Seek free medical services within your community

⇒ Find out if you qualify for Medicaid

⇒ See if any doctors in your area will take cash payments

Step 2: Verify every doctor is a "Valid Medical Source"

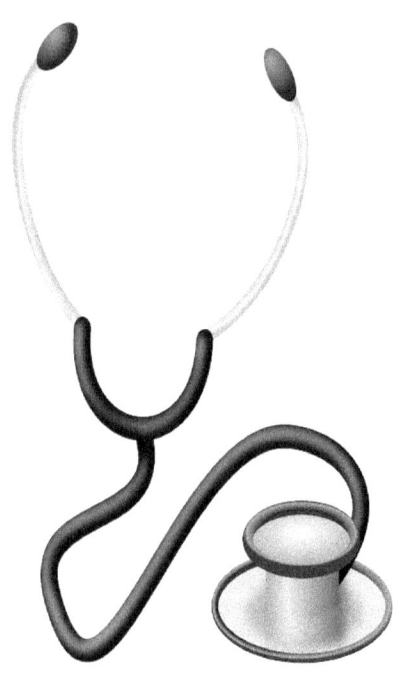

Acceptable medical source sounds complicated, but it is just a legal term to say your doctor is not a quack. They must be a licensed medical or osteopathic doctor, licensed or certified psychologist, licensed optometrist, licensed podiatrist, or qualified speech pathologist.

It's important to note, however, that just because your doctor says you are disabled does not guarantee that the SSA will agree. Your doctor's opinions must be supported by clinical observations, test results, or other supporting medical evidence which provide information about how your doctor determined the diagnosis and his assessment of your physical and mental capabilities.

It is also important that you have an ongoing relationship with the doctor, which means you go to see your doctor with a frequency which is consistent for your condition.

If the doctor is your treating doctor the SSA is required to defer to their medical opinion, unless they have a good reason to discount it. If they choose to discount the opinion they should give you information

Note:

If you do not have medical information about your disability because you have not seen a doctor, stop reading, shut this guide, and go to the doctor.

Review FAQ, "What if I cannot afford medical care?" if you have questions about getting medical care.

If the SSA gets your case and you have not seen a doctor they may send you to a consultative examiner for a consultative examination, but this generally does not help your case.

You DO NOT have to gather your own medical records. The SSA will do that for you FREE of CHARGE. You will have to provide information to the SSA about your doctors. If you have recent medical records, however, this can speed up your claim.

Step 3: Make sure your medical records clearly state why you are unable to work

For some reason claimants always seem confused about what they need to prove to win benefits. It's really quite simple. You need to prove that your health conditions are so severe they have completely eliminated your ability to work for at least 12 months continuous months.

The SSA has two different methods they will use to make a disability determination (which we will discuss later). Right now, it's important to make sure your medical files include information which specifically lists the physical and mental limitations you have to work five days per week for 8 hours each day.

Think about what tasks you are required to do each day. What tasks do you have difficulty performing because of your conditions? For example, if you have severe arthritis you may have difficulty typing or grasping small objects. A severe back condition may make it difficult to bend, stoop, or carry heavy objects.

Physical limitations can include:

⇒ The inability to walk, to stand, to crawl or to crouch
⇒ The inability to lift, to carry, to push, or to pull
⇒ The inability to hear or speak
⇒ The inability to manipulate objects with your hands

Mental Limitations can include:

⇒ Inability to concentrate and maintain attention for extended periods of time
⇒ Inability to adapt to new situations
⇒ Inability to remember short and simple instructions
⇒ Inability to Get along with co-workers

Non-traditional Treatments

The SSA will give little consideration to unproven, unscientific treatments. Common treatments that the SSA does not believe validate or support your claim can include megavitamin therapy, magnet therapy, juicing, aromatherapy, psychic diagnosis, rolfing, or applied kinesiology. More information about treatments that the SSA will not consider when evaluating your claim can be found at www.quackwatch.com

As medical technology changes and western doctors expand their notions about what may be valid treatments for different conditions, this information could change. Check with the Social Security Administration if you have questions about whether your treatment options are considered valid.

Step 3: Make sure your medical records clearly state why you are unable to work (cont.)

We will discuss this later when we review how to complete your application, but what your medical records need to provide is proof for the diagnosis, prognosis, and physical and mental limitations you list on your application.

Fore example, if you say, "I cannot sit more than two hours without getting up and walking around, and I cannot carry a box of paper (as required for my job) because of the severe pain it causes."

They will review what your doctor says on his medical reports. If they read that your doctor believes you not should not lift more than 5 lbs. or sit for more than 2 hours due to your severe back condition, this must be taken into consideration, but you will also need other objective types of medical evidence: laboratory tests, x-rays, clinical findings, blood tests, CT Scans, or MRIs.

Step 4: Verify your records are accurate, timely, and sufficient

If you want exhaustive information on this subject I would recommend reading Nolo's Guide to Social Security. It's a great book with an amazing amount of detail. I am just giving you the basics here.

With that said, your records should be timely, which means they are recent enough to be relevant to what you are claiming, accurate, describing your condition with standard and acceptable medical terms, and sufficient.

I have reviewed thousands of medical records over the last 8 years. One of the biggest issues I have seen, although this has gotten better with the initiative to move to electronic records, is that many claimant's records are not legible. If the SSA cannot read your records, they cannot use your records. It may be a good idea to request a copy of your medical records and review them.

BOTTOM LINE:

Doctors do not keep medical records with the purpose of helping you win SSDI benefits. The information they include generally is for treating your conditions. It's important to talk to your doctor and make sure your medical records aren't a jumbled mess and they clearly state your limitations to work.

Do not rely on your doctor to provide the right information on their own initiative. Get proactive. Talk to your doctor about your claim. Tell them what work activities you cannot perform. Have them make notes in your medical files. Demand the right tests to objectively document your health conditions. Be your own advocate!

Step 5: Make sure you have medical records that are related to your symptoms

We have talked about this a little bit, but you need to make sure your medical records clearly document how your disability is negatively impacting your ability to work and perform your daily activities.

Do you have trouble lifting a laundry basket?
Do you have someone helping you get in and out of the tub?
Can you still drive?
Do you take medication that makes it impossible to concentrate?
Can you do house or yard work?
Do you have severe pain? How often? What intensity? For how long?
What activities make your condition worse?
How much medication do you have to take? Dosage? Side-effects? Type?

Do you see what I am getting at? Your medical records need to provide EVIDENCE for your case, just as if you were proving another type of legal case.

If you get to your hearing and the judge asks you, "So Debbie, what do you do all day?" If you say, "Well sir, everyday I wake up and spend three hours tilling my garden, I go to the gym and work out, then I spend another couple of hours doing some heavy housework." The judge is likely to decide you are NOT disabled because your daily activity indicate you have the capacity to work.

NOTE:

The SSA will give little regard to what you say about your condition and symptoms if you have not DONE anything about them. For example, if you state that you have a severe back condition but you have not modified your daily activities or ever had to take prescription drug medications they may not believe you, especially if you do not have any other objective medical tests which prove your disability.

If you have a severe health condition follow your doctor's treatment plan, take your medications, document any activities you cannot perform, and keep a journal of all work activities that you cannot do due to your health condition.

Multiple attempts to perform less strenuous work or getting fired from a job because your condition does not allow you to do the work can also bolster your claim for disability.

STEP: 5

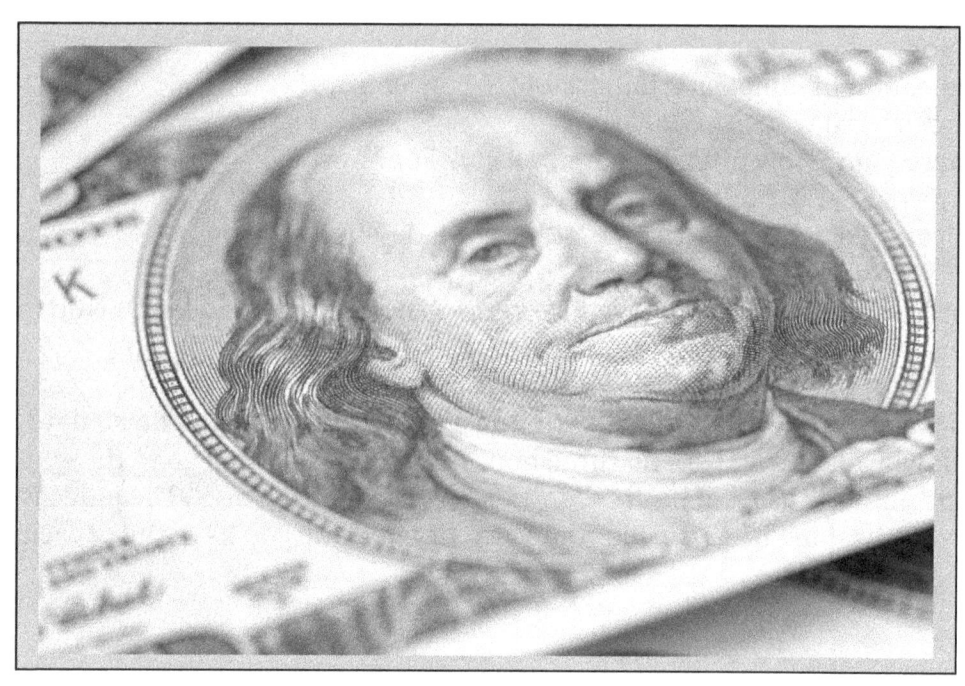

How do I apply for SSDI?

How do I apply for SSDI?

Step 1: Gather information for your SSDI Application

Now you may feel like you should be done with the process, but unfortunately, you are just starting. Assuming you have completed Steps 1 thru Step 4, it's time to file your SSDI application.

Before you start, however, you will need to gather all of the necessary information. The SSA provides a list at www.ssa.gov but the list is also provided below. Review the Disability Checklist BEFORE you to the SSA office, call the SSA, or start your online SSDI application.

FIRST THINGS FIRST:

Gather all or most of the information listed below to prepare to complete your SSDI application.

⇒ Birth and citizenship information
⇒ Name of your current and prior spouse (if the marriage lasted more than 10 years or ended in death)
⇒ Spouse(s) date of birth and SSN (optional)
⇒ Place of marriage
⇒ Name and birth dates of children who became disabled prior to the age of 22, or who are unmarried and under the age of 18 to 19 and still attending secondary school full time
⇒ US military service, including type of duty and branch service period date
⇒ Employer details for current year and prior 2 years. Go to www.ssa.gov/myaccount for employment information
⇒ Your employer's name
⇒ Employment start and end dates
⇒ Total earnings including wages and tips
⇒ Self-employment details for the current year and prior two years and business type and income
⇒ Direct deposit information including domestic bank (USA),
⇒ List of your medical condition(s)
⇒ Information about your doctors, healthcare professionals, hospitals, and clinics
⇒ Information about doctors, healthcare professionals, clinics, and hospitals
⇒ Names, addresses, phone numbers patient ID numbers, and dates of examination and treatments

Step 1: Gathering information for your SSDI Application (cont.)

⇒ Names and dates of medical tests and what doctor requested the tests
⇒ Names of medications (prescription and non-prescription) and reasons the medications were prescribed
⇒ Job history and date your medical condition began to affect your ability to work
⇒ Types of jobs (up to 5) that you have had in the past 15 years before you became unable to work
⇒ Dates you worked at those jobs, if available, and duties performed
⇒ Education and training, including the highest grade you completed and the date you completed it
⇒ Name of special job training, trade school and vocation school and date completed
⇒ Award letters, pay stubs, settlement agreements or other proof of any temporary or permanent workers' compensation type benefits you received
⇒ Your dog's name– just kidding, you don't need this!

You may not need to wait until you have every bit of this information to start your claim, but make sure you have most of it, especially if you are going to call the SSA or go to their office for SSA meeting.

All of the information which the SSA requests is used at some point in the application review or disability determination process.

Bottom Line:

The process is long, the SSA needs a heck of a lot of information. All the information gathered is used at some point in the disability application process. Some of the information is very important. We will talk about that later in the Guide.

Unfortunately, few people can help you. Your friends and family will generally know about as much as you do about the process. Don't count on help from the SSA either. The SSA representatives have thousands of claimants to help and will not have time to hold your hand.

But there is no reason to get discouraged. You already know more than you did. Knowing what information to include on your application is critical to winning benefits.

Don't worry. Keep reading and we will get through this together!!

Step 2: Choose how to apply for benefits

3 WAYS TO APPLY FOR BENEFITS

1. Go to the SSA office

This can be a total and utter beat down, especially if you have not made an appointment. Remember renewing your driver's license? Yeah, it's like that.

This option could be the best option, however, for claimants who need a little more face to face attention, help from the SSA, or who do not have the expertise to navigate the computer.

If you want to have a face-to-face interview make sure to call 1-800-772-1213 and schedule an interview. To facilitate the interview it's good to go to https://www.socialsecurity.gov/disability/ disability_starter_kits.htm and click on the Adult Disability Starter Kit. Printing and completing this worksheet and bringing it to the interview can really facilitate the interview process.

Attending the interview:
- You can bring a person to the interview.
- You can bring an interpreter to the interview.
- Do not bring children.
- Do not arrive late or they may cancel your appointment.
- Allow time to check-in and bring your ID.
- Do not tell long, detailed stories. Be accurate, precise, and concise with your answers to the questions

If you decide to go into the SSA office be aware that the SSA employee may be evaluating everything you do and say. If you say you have certain limitations but they see you perform tasks that contradict your statements, this might be noted in your file.

2. Apply over the phone

The beat down factor applying on the phone will be like going in to the office without an appointment. Over 2 million people apply for SSDI and SSI benefits each year, and most of them will call the SSA at some point in their lives. You do the math. Hold times can be significant.

The first time you call the SSA they will schedule an appointment time to call you back and complete the application over the phone. If you do decide to apply on the phone make sure you have reviewed the Disability Checklist and gathered all of your information.

3. Apply online at www.ssa.gov

This is by far the simplest and quickest way to apply, especially if you understand how to use a computer. The SSA site has improved over the years and is fairly easy to navigate. Note: not applicants will qualify to file online. Another benefits of this method is that you can log on, save your application, and return later.

Step 2: Choose how to apply for benefits (cont.)

To apply on-line:

1. Go to www.ssa.gov
2. Click on "Benefits" on the top of the screen
3. Select "Apply online for disability benefits"
4. Fill out the *Disability Benefit Application*
5. Answer the questions on the *Adult Disability Report*

To navigate through the on-line application process you can use the "Next" and "Previous" buttons on the top and bottom of each page. You can also move between sections with the tabs at the top of the screen. Avoid the "Enter" and "Back" buttons while in the Adult Disability Report.

You do not have to complete the entire report in one setting. You can click "Sign-off" to save your application and return to it at a later date. Make sure to write down your Reentry Number so you can access the form again.

Note:

As I stated before, applying online is by far the easiest and fastest way to apply for SSDI benefit. It also allows the claims representative to easily review your application and receive notification if any sections were not completed.

If you have not completed the application correctly or if you have left out pertinent information, the SSA representative will contact you for more information.

If you do not respond to the SSA or if they never get in contact with you, your application can be immediately denied.

The SSA gathers information on several forms:

1. The Adult Disability Report (Form SSA-3368-BK)
2. The Disability Benefit Application (Form SSA-16-F6)
3. Work History Report (Form SSA-3369-BK)
4. The Authorization to Disclose Information Form (SSA-827) which gives the SSA legal access to your medical records.

This form can be completed online as part of the Adult Disability Report, it can be printed and mailed to the SSA, or it can be taken to your local SSA office. The SSA cannot legally request your records until they have this form.

If you apply online some of these forms are grouped together. If you are filling out a hard-copy of any of the forms make sure you have the current version of the form (revision date is at the bottom left-hand corner). Always use blue or black ink and write legibly.

If you to go to a local SSA office to apply for SSDI benefits some offices will not accept hard-copies of the application but will have a SSA representative meet with you and type your answers directly into an online application.

Note: The SSA periodically updates their processes. These forms may be updated or eliminated.

I thought it was important to include the specifics for as many tasks as possible, but just know that things may have changed if you read this guide a year or two after it has been published.

Step 3: Completing your SSDI Application

The SSA asks a lot of questions. Winning benefits is about understanding WHY they are asking the question. Let's take look at what the SSA will ask you on the SSDI application and the SSA Disability Report.

Information about you

Make sure the SSA has correct information to contact you! If they can never contact you, they will dismiss your case.

Your illnesses, injuries or conditions and how they affect you

List EVERY condition that limits your ability to work, but make sure you have medical evidence to support every listed condition. We talked about this in Step 4. This is very important. Remember they are making their disability decision almost exclusively based on your medical information.

-Do not list medical conditions which do not limit your ability to work.
-Use the correct medical term which tells the official diagnosis (ex. Mitral valve prolapse is better than "heart issue")

Note:

Pay careful attention to what date you put as the "date you became unable to work." This date is referred to as your disability onset date. It may be modified later by the SSA, but assuming you are not working too much or making too much money and there is medical evidence that your condition started on this date, you may be entitled to back pay.

Work Activity

Work is classified by the SSA into different categories: sedentary, light, medium, and heavy. Each of these categories has very specific requirements. Work can also be classified as skilled work, semi-skilled work, and unskilled work.

Why does the SSA care? When determining whether you are disabled the SSA may use the information provided in this report to determine if you can work your current job or retrain for new work.

You do not need to list all of your employers, just the different job titles, job skills and requirements to perform the jobs.

If your condition does not meet a listing in the SSA Listing of Impairments (which we will discuss later), it is important to provide medical evidence that your impairment does not allow you to continue to work your current job or any job you have had in the past 15 years.

Step 3: Completing your SSDI Application (cont.)

Information about your medical records

You must provide accurate medical information. Nothing, and I mean nothing, will delay your SSDI application more than the SSA trying to request information from a doctor.

Providing inaccurate or incomplete information can lead to numerous phone calls with the SSA trying to reach you and clarify doctor contact information.

-Medical information should include laboratory test results and other objective medical evidence.
-Obtain the exact name, address, and phone numbers of treating sources, hospitals, and clinics
-Medical record numbers, clinic or admission numbers and dates of admission and discharge are also important

Medications

Include all medications you are taking and their side-effects. Medications can have severe side-effects which may make it difficult to perform work. For example, if you are taking medications which makes you drowsy and unable to operate heavy machinery this could reduce your ability to work a construction job.

Do not underestimate the importance of how a medication's severe side-effects can limit your ability to perform certain jobs.

Medical Tests

The SSA will expect for you to receive the proper medical testing. For example, if you have a severe back condition they will expect that you have had a MRI or CT scan.

It is important that you have had the proper medical tests. These tests provide objective medical evidence to support claims that you or your doctor make about your conditions.

Educational and Vocational Training

The SSA requests information about your educational background because they will assume that a highly educated claimant will have a greater chance of retraining for new work than a high school drop-out. Claimants with vocational training may also have a higher chance of returning to work.

Information about your spouse and children

If you qualify for SSDI benefits and you are married and have children, in some cases, your spouse and dependent children may also qualify for auxiliary benefits.

If the SSA does not know you are married or have children your qualifying family members will not receive their auxiliary benefits, and that's money you've lost.

If you did not include information about your family on your application be sure to contact the SSA. Additionally, if you have a life change (i.e., you get married, a spouse dies, you have a baby, or you get divorced, contact the SSA and notify them of the family change).

Step 3: Completing your SSDI Application (cont.)

Employment Information

The SSA must verify you have sufficient work credits to be considered insured for SSDI benefits. If you are not sure about whether you qualify for SSDI, if you would like to track your earnings, or you do not believe the SSA has your full earning record, go to www.ssa.gov/myaccount to verify your employment information.

After you submit your SSDI application:

If you apply for SSDI online you will be given a reference number to return to your application, if needed. If you decide to apply by sending hard copy forms to the SSA make sure you keep copies of all the information you send.

You can check the status of your disability application within five days after an online submission by going to www.ssa.gov and clicking on the drop down menu "Benefits." Click on the "Disability" option on the menu, and then click the "Check Application Status" button in the middle of the page.

After you submit your application to the SSA either online, by mail, or over the phone, the local SSA will review it. If you meet the nonmedical requirements they will send it to the DDS office for a full medical review.

You may receive calls from the SSA at any point in the process. Be patient. If you do not meet the nonmedical requirements you will receive a denial immediately, generally within a month or two. If you meet the nonmedical requirements the DDS may take up to 6 months to review the application, although the SSA states that it should take around 90 days.

Tips for completing the application:

⇒ Do not overstate what you can do
⇒ Do not understate the severity of your symptoms
⇒ Keep your answers brief and to the point
⇒ Presume you are evaluating your worst day
⇒ Remember that you are providing information about activity you can do on a sustained basis (5 days/per week, 8 hours/day)
⇒ Focus on the frequency, duration, and severity of your symptoms (e.g., pain, fatigue, and limitations)
⇒ Include any psychological issues that may keep you from working
⇒ List every condition that affects your ability to work

IMPORTANT:

SSDI fraud is a crime. If you provide information which is intentionally inaccurate and receive benefits you do not deserve, you could be charged with fraud.

STEP: 6

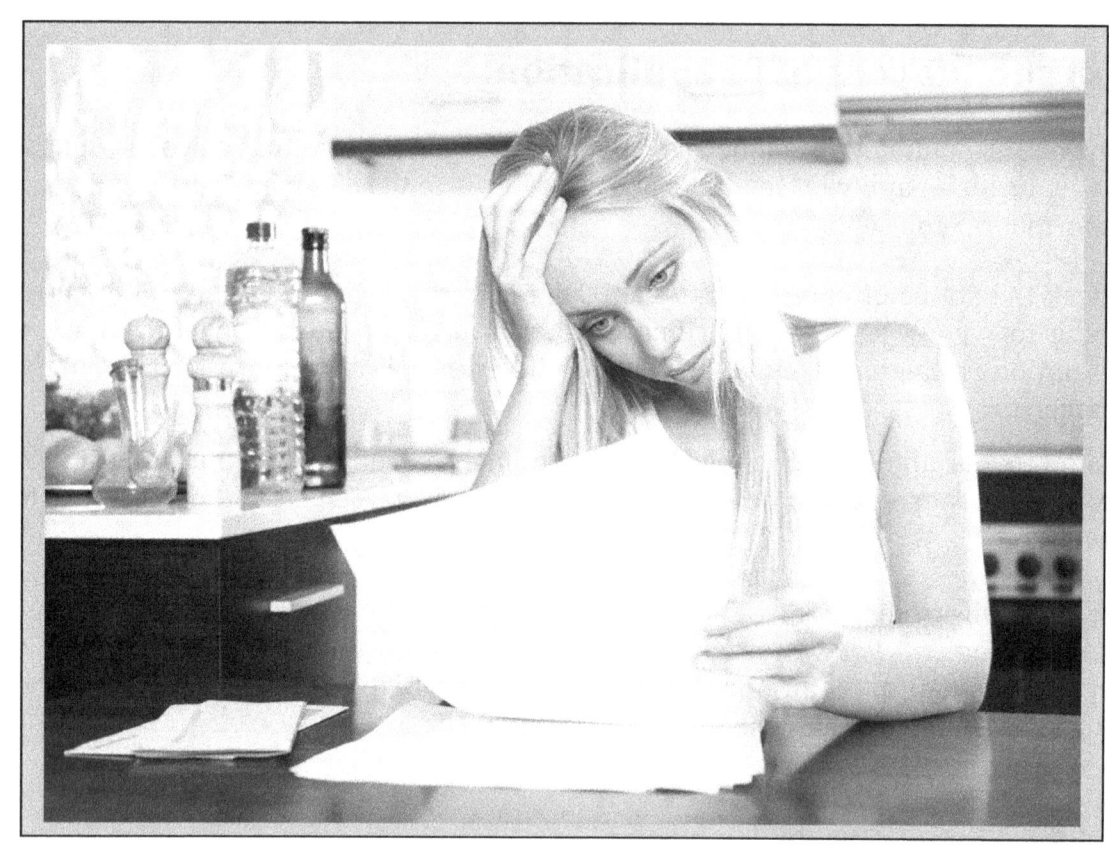

What do I need to understand about the SSDI application process?

What do I need to understand about the SSDI application process?

Step 1: Understand where your application is in the SSDI approval process

Disability Application Process

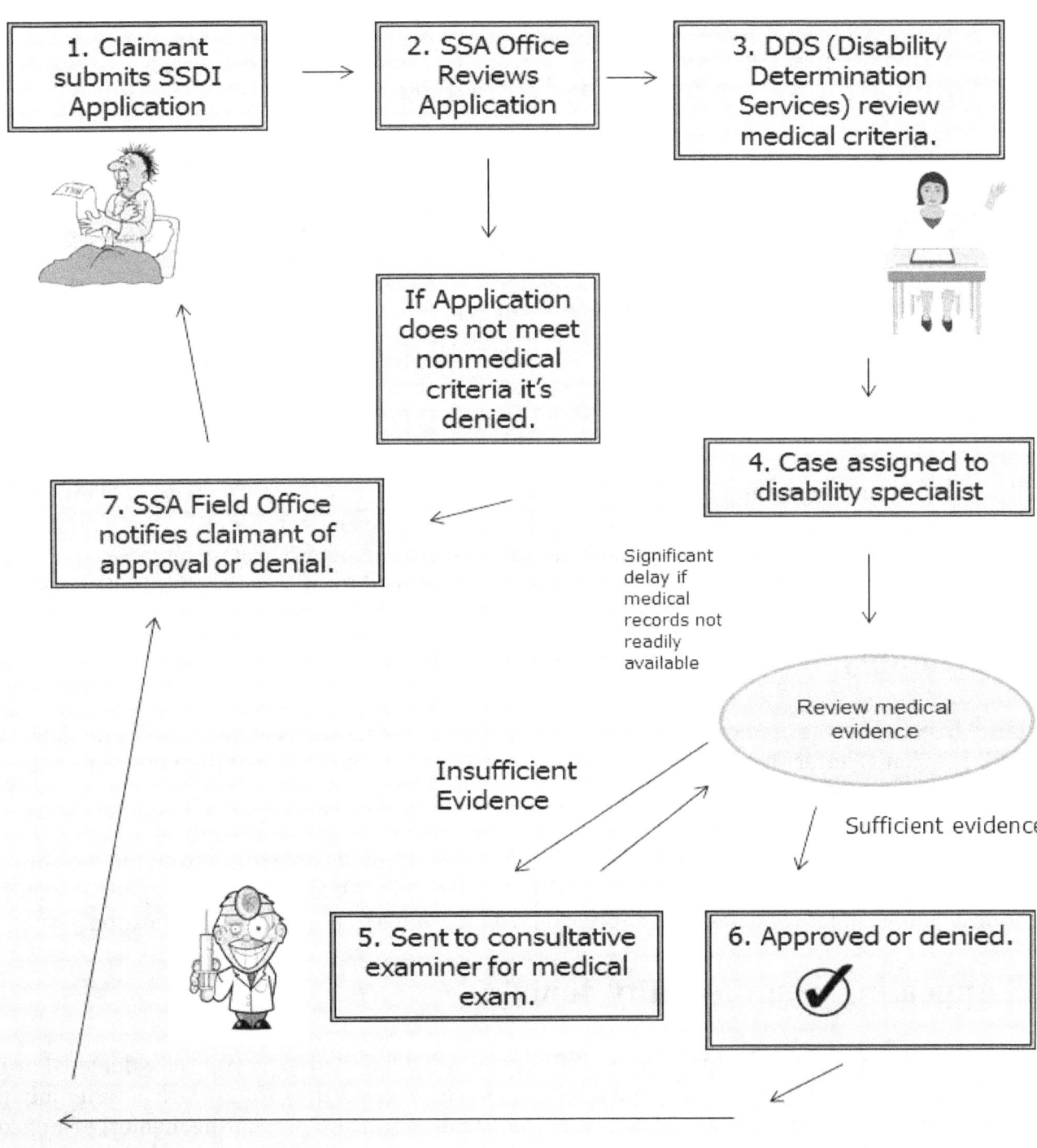

Step 2: Understand what happens to your SSDI application at every step in the process

1. Submit your SSDI application to the SSA

If you have met the non-medical requirements for SSDI, the SSDI application is sent to the appropriate Disability Determinations Services Offices (DDS) for review. The SSA states that it can take 90 to 120 days for the Disability Determinations Services Office to review the claim and make a disability determination. Assume it will take 3 to 5 months. Up to 70% of initial disability applications are denied.

2. Application reviewed at the DDS Office

The amount of time needed for a review at the DDS office can vary depending on whether or not the DDS has all of the necessary medical records or whether you have to visit a consultative examiner. The DDS will request information from each doctor, hospital, and clinic you listed on your application/Disability Report. You will be given the name and number of your DDS examiner. The SSA would only like you to contact the DDS examiner if you have new medical information that they need to process your claim, if you believe they need help getting your medical records, or it has been more than 4 months and you have not received any information about your case.

3. Disability benefits approved by the DDS

If the DDS approves the application you will receive a Notice of Award. The local field office will, however, ensure you continue to meet the nonmedical requirements prior to issuing the letter. Note: The SSA does not pay for the first 5 months you are disabled. This is referred to as the "5 month waiting period." Retroactive benefits are also not paid for this 5 month waiting period.

4. Disability benefits denied by the DDS

If the DDS denies the application they will notify the local SSA office who will send a denial letter to you. The denial letter should detail why your benefits were denied and outline the steps you can take to appeal your denial.

This process is discussed later in the book, but in general, you have 60 days from the date of the denial letter (really 65 because the SSA allows 5 days for mailing), to submit your appeal. If you miss your deadline, unless you have a great reason, you will have to file another application.

5 Appealing your disability denial

Whether or not you should appeal your SSDI denial will depend on why you were denied. For instance, claimants who have been denied because the SSA stated they could work another job may be able to appeal their medical denial by filing a reconsideration and presenting medical evidence that they cannot retrain for new work.

Step 3: Understand how the SSA makes their disability determination

Now that you understand the application process, let's discuss the disability decision making process. The first question most claimants ask about the disability process is, "How the heck does the SSA make their disability decision?"

It's easy to assume the SSA makes their disability decisions arbitrarily. Believe it or not, however, there is a method to the madness. It is called the 5 Step Sequential Evaluation Process. Let's break it down.

FIVE STEP SEQUENTIAL EVALUTION PROCESS

When the SSA gets your SSDI application they will ask five questions. Depending on the answer, they will either find you disabled and award you SSDI benefits, or they will go to the next step.

You can be disabled if, after the relevant questions are asked, they find any of the following to be true:

-Your condition meets a listing on the SSA Listing of Impairments
-You are not able to work any job you have previously worked in the last 15 years
-You are not able to adjust to new work

Let's take a look at the five questions.

QUESTION 1:
Are you working too much or making too much money?

If you are working too much or making too much money, you are not disabled. The SSA calls work at this level substantial gainful activity (SGA). The amount you can earn changes periodically. In 2016, the amount is $1,130 per month in gross earnings for non- blind individuals. If you are making more than this amount each month, you are NOT disabled.

You can also be determined disabled if you are working too much. I touched on this before, but if you perform 40 hours of volunteer work each week the SSA would consider you not disabled, even though you are not making a profit. The SSA's assumption is that if you can do 40 hours of volunteer work each week, you can do 40 hours of work for pay.

If you make less than this amount or do not perform substantial work, the SSA proceeds to the next

Step 3: Understand how the SSA makes their disability determination (cont.)

QUESTION 2:
Is your condition severe?

A severe condition is one which will last at least 12 continuous months and interferes with basic work-related activities.

Basic work-related activities include physical actions such as lifting, carrying, sitting, and standing (the activities that you SHOULD have listed on your application that you were having trouble performing due to your condition).

Basic work-related activities can also include mental activities, such as your ability to understand and carry out instructions, make work-related judgments, and deal with a work routine.

QUESTION 3:
Does your condition meet or exceed a Listing?

Everybody loves lists, and the SSA has a list of the most common health conditions and their corresponding symptoms which they consider automatically disabling. This list is referred to as the "Blue Book" or the SSA Listing of Impairments. If your condition and symptoms are on this list or they are as severe as a condition on this list, you are disabled. If not, proceed to the next step.

If the SSA proceeds to step 4 they will assess your residual functional capacity to work. In plain language this means your maximum ability to work and perform work-related tasks for 8 hours per day/5 days per week.

They will also determine your limitations and your restrictions. Both of these factors are considered when they determine your physical and mental functional capacity to work.

It's a lot of SSA jargon, but the bottom line is they are trying to find out what work you can do given your medical condition(s) and the related symptoms.

If you want to review the list just google SSA Listing of Impairments. There is a child and adult list. Make sure you look at the Adult Listing.

QUESTION 4:
Can you perform past relevant work?

The SSA reviews your residual functional capacity to work and compares it to the job requirements

Step 3: Understand how the SSA makes their disability determination (cont.)

of your past relevant work. In other words, do you have the remaining capacity to do any full-time job you have done in the last 15 years?

(At this step the SSA does not consider your age, education, employability, or whether past relevant work exists in the national economy.)

Note: You are responsible for providing information to the SSA that you have an impairment which does not allow you to perform past relevant work.

If you cannot perform past work, the SSA will find that you are disabled. If not, they will proceed to step five.

QUESTION 5:
Can you retrain for new work?

Now, it really gets fun. The SSA now has the burden of proving that although you cannot work any past job, you can retrain and work another job which exists in significant numbers in the national economy.

At this step the SSA will consider not only your impairment, but also your age, your education, and previous work experience.

The process to make this decision is based on Special Medical Profiles as well as Medical Vocational Guidelines (referred to as "The Grids"). Suffice it to say this is complicated. Go to www.SSA.gov and search for SSA's Sequential Evaluation Process for Assessing Disability if you need more exciting information on this process.

If the SSA decides you can make an adjustment to other work, they will find you NOT disabled. If they decide you cannot make an adjustment to other work, they will find you disabled.

NOTE:

There are hundreds, if not thousands, of articles online about Meeting a Listing or proving that you are disabled according to the requirements outlined by the SSA. If you need more details than what I have provided above get online and start reading!!

Step 4: Understand what it means to "Meet a Listing"

Meeting or equaling a listing is one of the easiest ways to qualify for SSDI benefits, assuming you've met the nonmedical requirements SSDI (i.e., not making too much money, having enough work credits, and meeting the age requirements).

Let's talk a little more about what it really means to "meet or equal a listing."

Meeting or equaling a listing =

Having a condition and corresponding symptoms listed on the SSA Listing of Impairments.

OR

Having a condition and corresponding symptoms which are as
SEVERE as a condition on the listing,

OR you don't meet the criteria but the medical findings of your case have the same meaning as the criteria,

OR you have a combination of impairments which if taken together, are as severe as a listing.

The Listing is divided into an Adult Listing and a Child Listing so make sure you look at the right listing. The Listing is currently divided into 14 major body systems and further divided within each section (periodic updates are done).

For most applicants I'd recommend reviewing the Listing (google SSA Listing of Impairments) and seeing what you need to prove to meet the listing, but as mentioned before, without a medical degree you are going to have to do a lot of research to fully grasp what the heck you are reading.

One great resource ii you are really curious about all of this is Nolo's Guide to Social Security Disability. They dedicate almost half of their book to breaking down each system and the corresponding symptoms.

You can also discuss your case with your doctor or lawyer. They should know more about whether your case meets or equals a listing.

One thing I will mention here, however, is that just like you should not expect too much from the SSA, I would not expect too much from your doctor.

A doctor may be willing to fill out a short form outlining what they believe are your limitations to work (this form is referred to as a Residual Functional Capacity form or RFC form), but I would not expect them to help you too much through this process.

I definitely would not hand them the disability application and say, "Here, can you feel this out for me?"

They are likely to laugh.

NOTE:

There are lawyers or disability advocates who will help you file your application for SSDI. Not all of them will, but if you need help you could call a few and find out your options.

After you have submitted your application to the SSA, now it is time to wait. It could take up to five months to hear back from them. Generally, however, they will make their decision within 90 days.

When you do get your response, if you get an approval, you are done. If not, go to the next section and find out how to appeal the denial.

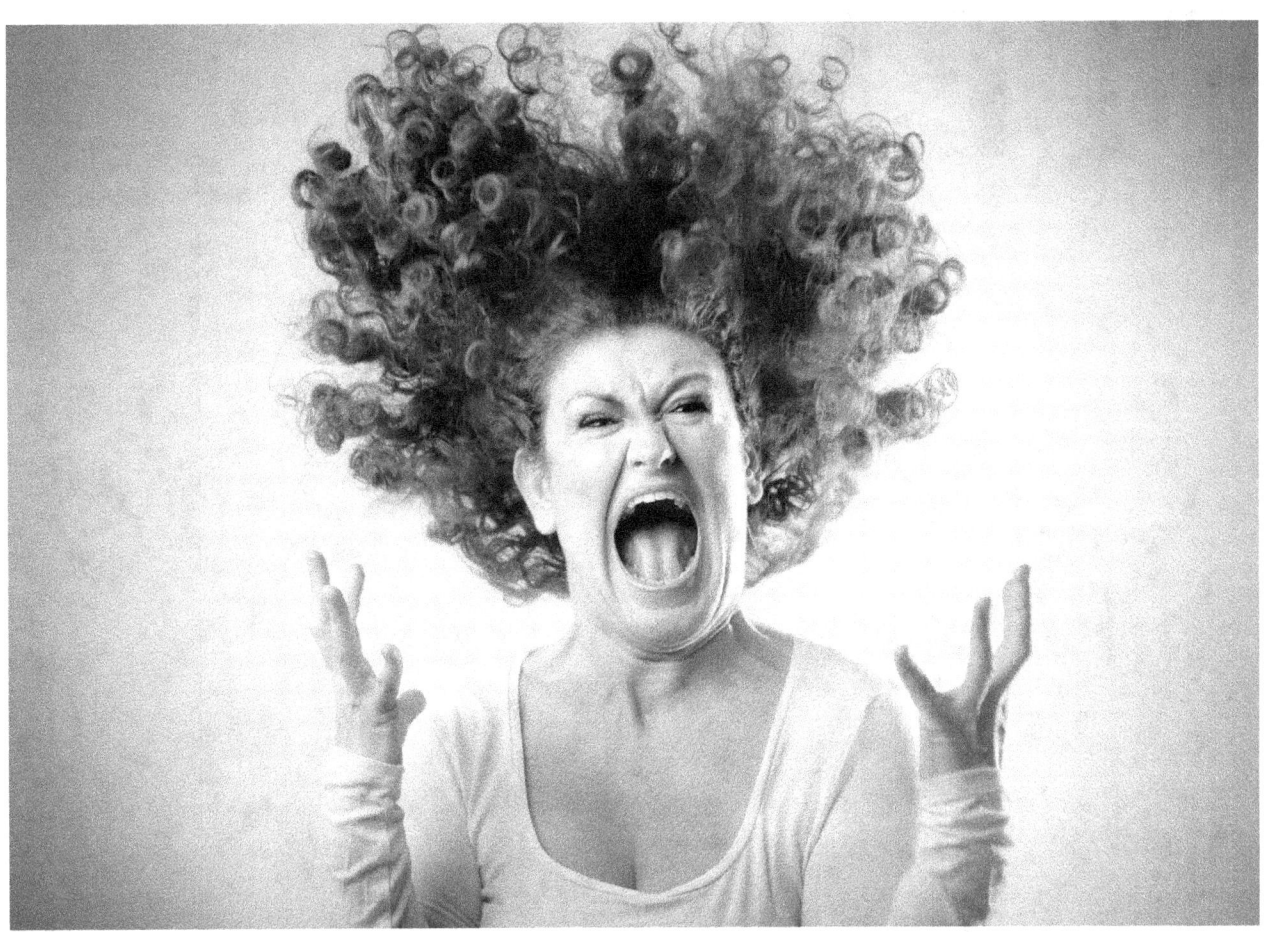

If you feel like this woman, don't panic. Remember the following:

⇒ Meeting a Listing is the fastest and easiest way to win benefits the first time you apply. Unfortunately, the Listing of Impairments is difficult to understand for the average claimant.

⇒ Review the Listing of Impairments BEFORE you apply.

⇒ Talk to your doctor about your conditions and symptoms and whether they meet a listing.

⇒ Make sure you have enough medical evidence to prove your condition meets or exceeds a listing.

⇒ Make sure you either submit the medical evidence to the SSA or they have the right information to request the medical evidence from your doctors.

⇒ If your condition does not meet a listing make sure your medical evidence clearly states the limitations you have to perform your current job and past jobs.

⇒ If your condition does not meet a listing make sure your medical evidence clearly states your limitations to do other less strenuous jobs (this information is critical to prove to the SSA that you cannot retrain for other work).

⇒ If all of this is really confusing consider talking to a disability lawyer and find out if they think you have a strong case.

STEP: 7

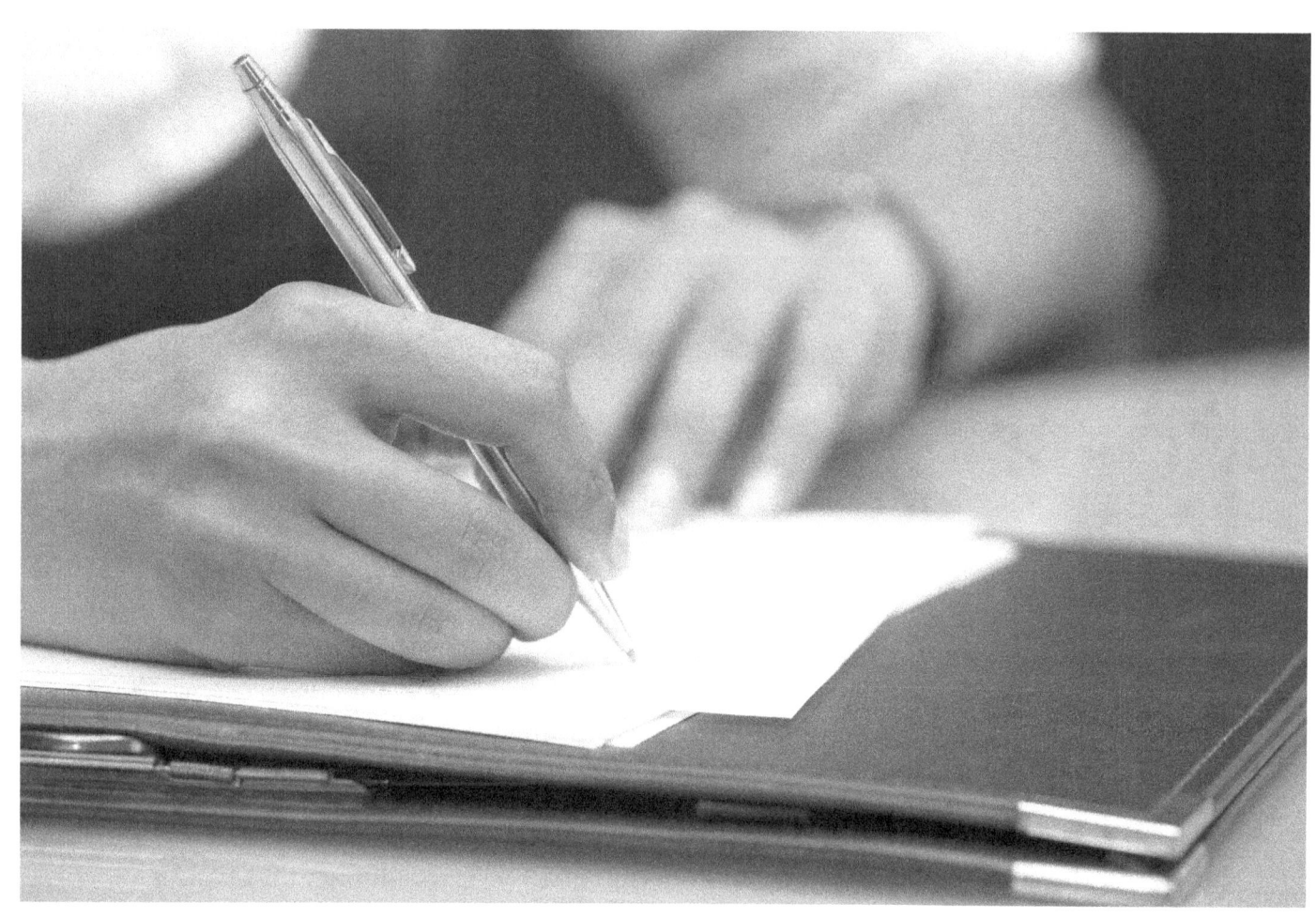

How do I appeal my SSDI denial?

How do I appeal my SSDI denial?

Most SSDI claims are denied. In fact, on average 70% of disability claims are denied at the application level. What do you do if you are denied?

1. Review your denial letter and determine why your case was denied. Not all denials can be easily appealed.
2. If you do not have sufficient work credits, and the SSA calculated your credits correctly, you will not qualify for SSDI benefits. Talk to the SSA and find out if you can qualify for SSI benefits.
3. If the SSA states that your condition is not severe, you can retrain for new work, or your condition is short-term, you may be able to provide additional medical evidence to challenge the denial.

All appeals must be made within 60 days from the date of the denial letter. Miss the appeal deadline without a good reason and you will have to apply again and start from the very beginning, and NOBODY wants that.

Another option is to file a new application. This is not recommended. A hearing, which is the second appeal in most states, generally gives you the best chance to win benefits. Applying over and over again does not get you to the hearing.

Do I need a lawyer to appeal my disability decision?

No one has to hire a lawyer, but I will say what I have been telling claimants for years. Not hiring a lawyer can be a bit like cutting your own hair, you can do it, but you may not be happy with the results.

Just because you CAN do something does not mean you should.

Hiring a lawyer will cut into your benefit payout, but disability lawyers only get paid if they win your case. If they win, they are paid 25% of your back pay up to a maximum of $6,000.

Not all claimants will have that much back pay, but almost all claimants have some back pay simply because it can take over a year to have your hearing scheduled.

So with that said, if you have no interest in learning about the disability process, what you need to prove to win, how you need to argue your case before the judge– close this guide and call a lawyer and let them file the appeal paperwork for you.

Is a lawyer worth the money?

This is a tough question. If you have applied multiple times for SSDI and you have waited months for benefits and the lawyer is able to swoop in and help you win at your SSDI hearing, well, you may have lost $6,000, but you won on-going monthly benefits until you reach your full retirement age, you go back to work, or the SSA determines you are no longer disabled.

If your disability lawyer is worthless, and yes there are some who are, they do not work on your case, they come unprepared to the hearing, and you lose...well, you are back to square one BUT you won't owe the lawyer any money!

Step 1: Filing an SSDI Appeal

Assuming you do not go back to work, file a new application, hire a lawyer, or do nothing, you have 60 days from the date of the denial letter to file your appeal. In most states the first appeal is called a reconsideration. Other states, however, allow claimants to immediately request a hearing.

1. Filing a reconsideration

If you have received a medical denial you can appeal the decision online by going to the SSA website at www.ssa.gov, choosing "Benefits," choosing "Disability," then choosing "Appeal our Recent Medical Decision."

Medical decisions can also be appealed by completing:

=Request for Reconsideration (Form SSA-561)
=Disability Report - Appeal (Form SSA-3441)
=Authorization to Disclose Information to the SSA (Form SSA-827)

If your application is denied for nonmedical reasons you can contact your local Social Security Office to request a technical review. You may also call the SSA at their toll-free number, 1-800-772-1213, to request an appeal.

After you submit your reconsideration, it can take up to 90 days to find out if you have been approved or denied. If denied, you have 60 days from the date of the letter to file another appeal for the hearing. Unfortunately, up to 80% of reconsiderations are denied.

2. Requesting a SSDI Administrative Hearing

Most states require a reconsideration appeal prior to requesting a hearing. For states that eliminate the hearing or if your case is denied a second time, you can file for a hearing by taking these steps:

Option 1:
Filing online

Go to www.socialsecurity.gov/forms and clicking on Appeal a Recent Medical Decision, which takes you to the online process.

Option 2:
Complete three forms

These forms can be downloaded by visiting: www.socialsecurity.gov/forms/ha-501.html

> Form HA-501- Request for Hearing by Administrative Law Judge,
> SSA-3441, Disability Report - Appeal
> SSA-827, Authorization to Disclose Information to SSA

Filing an SSDI Appeal (cont.)

Option 3:
Call the SSA and tell them you would like to appeal your denial.

Most likely the SSA will direct you to one of the processes described on the previous page. Do not request for them to send you the hard copy forms to appeal, this is a waste of your time If you need help appealing your denial you could also go into the local SSA office and talk to a SSA representative.

If you hire a lawyer you will need to complete form SSA-1696, Appointment of Representative, which notifies the SSA you have hired a lawyer. Your lawyer will complete your appeal for you.

What information do I include on my appeal when they ask for a explanation?

- List any medical sources which provided information which were not reviewed
- Notify the SSA that the medical decision they used to make the decision was not the condition you identified or described
- Notify the SSA that you listed more conditions than they considered based on their denial
- Provide information about how your physical or mental limitations are more severe than the SSA believes
- List all new medical sources that were not included at the time of the first application
- List all new medical conditions you now suffer from
- List all new medications that affect your ability to work

How long will I have to wait for my hearing?

There's no way to sugar-coat this; you are going to be waiting for your hearing months, if not years. Unfortunately, average wait times for hearings vary by region. Review the FAQ, "How long will I have to wait for my SSDI hearing?" for more information about the average wait times for your region. It's important to file the reconsideration, however, and get to this point. Your chance of getting approved for SSDI increases substantially at the hearing level. Make sure you take the right steps and understand what you need to prove. Just a bit further, I promise!

Considerations:

- ⇒ *Most claimants are denied at the application and reconsideration levels.*
- ⇒ *Claimants have the best chance of winning benefits at the hearing level.*
- ⇒ *Hiring a lawyer to present your case before a judge is generally a good idea at the hearing level.*
- ⇒ *Claimants generally have to wait more than one year to have their hearing scheduled.*
- ⇒ *If you lose at your hearing most lawyers suggest starting again from the beginning rather than appealing your case to the Appeals Council.*

STEP: 8

What do I do to get ready for my hearing?

What do I do to get ready for my hearing?

GOOD NEWS!!

Your SSDI administrative hearing is your best chance to win SSDI benefits. Let me say that again, your hearing is your best chance to win benefits. You have waited up to two years and now you have the opportunity to make your case before an administrative law judge who has the authority to decide your case.

Five words:

DO NOT MESS IT UP.

Step 1: Talk to a disability lawyer

As I mentioned before, this is totally optional. Many claimants win without lawyers, and many claimants lose with them. All I will say is this: I have dealt with a lot of claimants and there are not many who can adequately argue their case or understand what they are arguing. If you can, that's awesome! I wish you the best!

Step 2: Make sure your medical evidence is up to date and you have recently seen a doctor.

Sometimes you may have to wait up to 2 years for your hearing. Many claimants have conditions which get progressively worse. You want the judge to understand your current condition, not what it might have been two years ago.

Additionally, make sure during this time you continue to receive medical care, you follow your doctor's treatment plan, and the SSA has received recent medical information which will support your case.

Before the SSDI administrative hearing you should do the following:

Ensure the judge has all recent and updated medical reports.
Make sure to have evidence to counter all claims you cannot work.
Have your lawyer submit a brief (a short document stating your case and relevant medical information to support your case) to the administrative law judge prior to the hearing.

What do I have to do to get ready for my hearing ? (cont.)

Step 3: Understand the disability hearing process.

This is an especially important step if you do not hire a lawyer. Either way it's a good idea to make sure you know the types of questions the judge will ask, the pros and cons of your case, and how to prove you are disabled and cannot work.

If you have hired a lawyer they will do most of the talking at the hearing, and they should provide evidence to support your case.

Step 4: Keep up with your SSDI case

There is no need to badger the SSA or your lawyer, but it's not a bad idea to check in with all parties every three months or so to ensure your case is on track and no one has tried to contact you for information.

Step 5: Prepare for your hearing

1. Review your file, your record, and the evidence for your case

Every disability claimant has a file. If you have a lawyer they will have a copy of your file. If not, get a copy and look through it.

2. Make sure you have a full list of your medications

Not only do you need a full list of conditions, you also need medical records to substantiate each condition. For example, if you say you have a back issue, you will need medical tests, lab tests, medical notes, etc. which support your claim.

3. Find out if there will be a vocational and medical expert at your hearing

Review what roles each expert will play in your hearing. Understand how to counter any claims from the vocational expert that you can work other jobs in the national economy. They will most likely state you can retrain for new work and list jobs they think you can do. You need to be able to give specific symptoms, limitations, etc. that would make it impossible for you to do those jobs.

3. Understand the hearing procedures

This is not an episode of *Law and Order* and you will not be in front of a court room full of people, but you do need to understand how the hearing is held.

4. Be courteous, honest, and pay attention to each party as they testify

What do I have to do to get ready for my hearing ? (cont.)

Step 6: Understand what will happen at the hearing

As I mentioned before, the SSDI administrative hearing is not like an episode of *Law and Order* with Jack McCoy badgering you on the witness stand.

Most likely it will be held in a small room. A judge, court reporter, your attorney (if you hire one), the vocational expert, and the medical expert will be present. The judge will begin by asking you a series of questions about your background, your work history, your medical condition(s), and your daily activities.

Your lawyer may also answer a series of questions about your case. Generally, if a vocational expert (VE) is present, the vocational expert will testify about work they believe you can do given your current health care conditions and your limitations.

The VE will provide the job titles, the job codes, and the number of jobs in the area for the employment they believe you could do in your area (information they have gathered from the Dictionary of Occupational Titles (DOT), County business patterns published by the Bureau Census, and the Occupational Outlook Handbook published by Bureau of Labor Statistics).

Your attorney will have an opportunity to counter their claims. If you do not have a lawyer you should be ready to counter claims with medical evidence that you cannot work the jobs they suggest.

For example, if they state you can work as a staff assistant, which is a sedentary job, you will need to provide evidence that you cannot. Exertional limitations that may eliminate the ability to perform sedentary work include: the inability to lift up to 10 pounds, the required use of a hand-held device to walk, the need to keep your legs elevated, the inability to sit for six hours out of a eight hour day, etc. You see what I am getting at? You will need medical evidence to eliminate sedentary work as an option.

Note: The ability to provide evidence that you cannot do the jobs they suggest is generally the most critical part of the disability hearing.

At the conclusion of the hearing the judge may make a statement. At some hearings the judge may make statements that sound favorable for your case. Do not make any assumptions. The decision of the judge are not final until they provide a written statement documenting their decision.

Steps to follow at the hearing:

- Do not exaggerate your medical problems
- Do not minimize your symptoms
- Answer all of your questions honestly
- Do not bring up unsolicited information which can hurt your case
- Do not give vague answers. For example, if you have migraines do not say I have migraines and they hurt. Say, instead, "I have migraines four days per week. They last for 2 hours, and I have to go to bed due to the throbbing pain."

SSDI Appeals Process

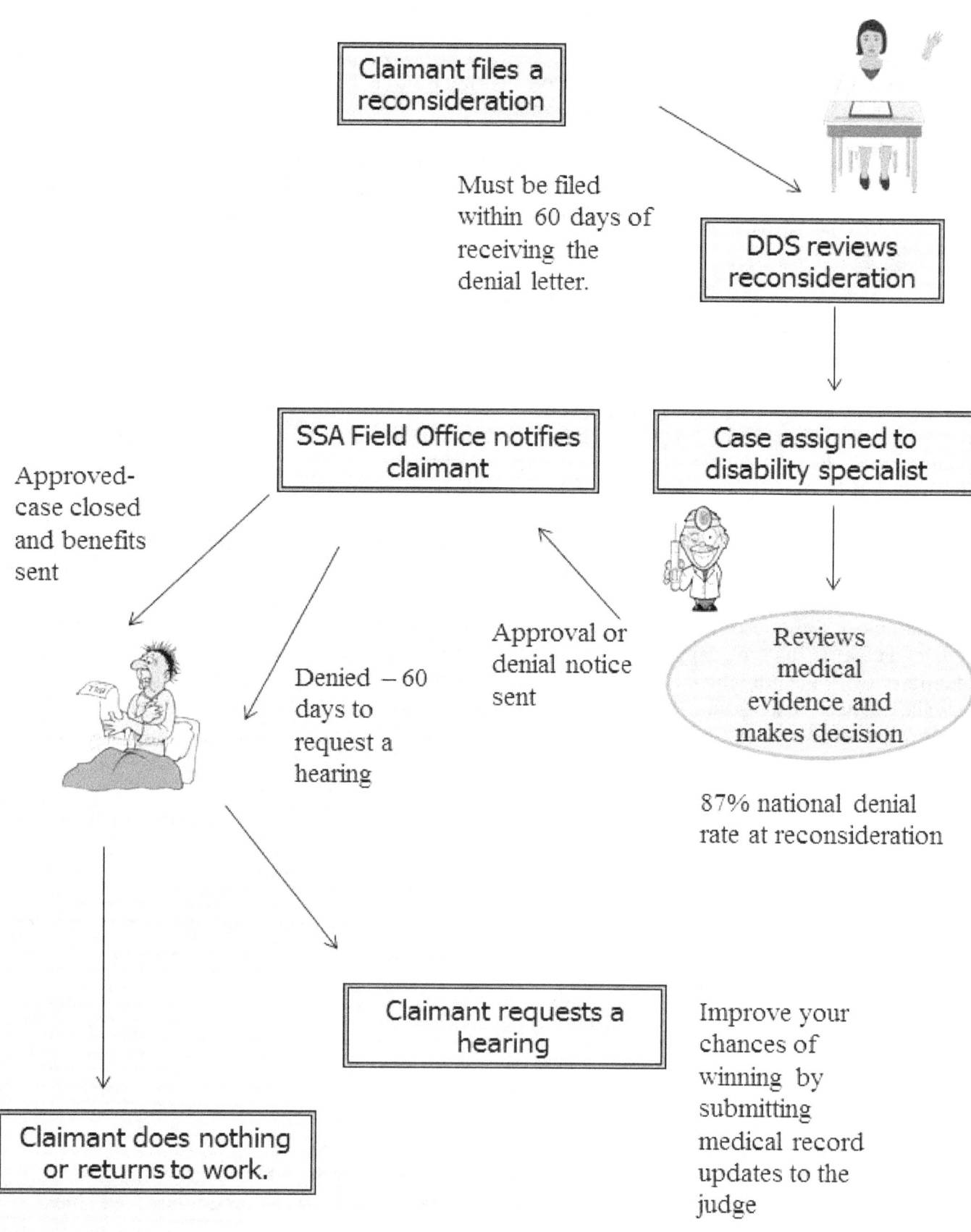

Claimant files a reconsideration

Must be filed within 60 days of receiving the denial letter.

DDS reviews reconsideration

SSA Field Office notifies claimant

Case assigned to disability specialist

Approved-case closed and benefits sent

Approval or denial notice sent

Reviews medical evidence and makes decision

Denied – 60 days to request a hearing

87% national denial rate at reconsideration

Claimant requests a hearing

Improve your chances of winning by submitting medical record updates to the judge

Claimant does nothing or returns to work.

Understand what happens after the hearing

Hopefully, after the hearing you are approved and receive notification about your benefits from the court within a few months. If you are approved you will receive an Awards Letter which details the month of your first payment and the payment amount.

If you receive another denial, you can file another request to have your case heard by the Appeals Council. The Appeals Council may decide to review your case, remand it back to the administrative judge, or review it and issue a new decision.

Unfortunately, most disability lawyers will advise against appealing to the Appeals Council given the low probability that they will review your case and issue a favorable ruling. Most lawyers suggest filing a new application.

If you get to this point I am very sorry. You are looking at several really bad options: submitting a new SSDI claim and starting the process again or filing a case with the Appeals Council and waiting months or years for a decision, assuming they review your case at all.

Unfortunately, many disability lawyers will not take a case at the Appeals Council level if they have not been working on the case from the beginning.

It's important to do your best to win at the hearing; that's why I suggest hiring a lawyer.

Conclusion

By far the most common question asked by a claimant is, "When will I get my benefits?" So I will close with this question.

You may never receive your SSDI benefits. There are a variety of reasons for this: you may not have enough work credits, you may have a short-term condition, you may be able to work, you may be working too many hours, or you may be making too much money when you apply for benefits.

If you do qualify, however, and you are approved at the application level, it could take up to 90 days to review your case. Add in another month or two to process you payment and you're already up to four months of potential wait time.

If you have to appeal your case through a reconsideration that can add 90 additional days. (if you are lucky). If you are denied at the reconsideration level you can appeal your denial through an Administrative Hearing, but that can add up to 2 years onto your SSDI disability case as you wait months and months to get a disability hearing. What this means for most claimants is that they are going to wait potentially months or even years to win benefits.

What this means for you is that you need to do everything you can to win the first time you apply. The best way to do that is to follow the steps outlined in GIMME MY SSA DISABILITY!. Assuming you meet the nonmedical requirements for SSDI, following the steps outlined in this Guide should substantially increase your chances of winning benefits the first time you apply.

Frequently Asked Questions

List of Frequently Asked Questions

1. How long do I have to wait for my SSDI hearing?
2. What can I expect at my SSDI hearing?
3. When do I appeal my SSDI hearing?
4. Do I need a lawyer to file a SSDI appeal?
5. How far back will I be paid SSDI?
6. How is SSDI different than unemployment benefits?
7. How long does it take to file my SSDI application?
8. How long will a SSDI appeal take with a lawyer?
9. What does a lawyer do for the money?
10. How much will the disability lawyer be paid?
11. How many work credits will I need for SSDI?
12. Is SSDI only for those with a permanent disability?
13. What if my condition improves?
14. Denied twice can a lawyer help?
15. Why won't a lawyer take my disability case?
16. Why was I denied SSDI?
17. How can I generate work credits for SSDI?
18. Can I borrow work credits from a spouse?
19. No work credits but I cannot work. What are my options?
20. Can I file a reconsideration on my own?
21. How do you file your own reconsideration?
22. What is the difference between SSDI and SSI?
23. Unemployment benefits are gone should I file for SSDI?
24. What do I need to know about SSDI before I apply?
25. I sent my application to the SSA why have I not heard from them?
26. Who will request my medical records?
27. Will I get medical insurance if I qualify for SSDI?
28. Can I work part-time and get SSDI?
29. Can my wife and children get SSDI benefits?
30. SSA says my disability started after my date last insured (DLI) what does this mean?
31. What if I cannot afford medical care?
32. What if I go back to work before the DDS makes the medical decision?

1. How long do I have to wait for my SSDI hearing?

One thing you can count on is the inefficiency of the federal government. If you are waiting for a SSDI it's time to grab your coffee, sit back, put your feet up, and get ready to wait.

If you have requested a hearing you are waiting for the Office of Disability Adjudication and Review (ODAR) to schedule a hearing before an Administrative Law Judge (ALS). There is only one hearing location with an average wait time of less than 12 months.

Amount of days on average for a hearing to be scheduled for each of the regions in the U.S:

Region I (Massachusetts, New Hampshire, Connecticut, Maine and Rhode Island) 354 days.
Region II (New York, Puerto Rico and New Jersey) 484 days
Region III (Pennsylvania, Virginia, West Virginia, Maryland, and Washington DC) 348 days Region IV (Georgia, Alabama, North Carolina, South Carolina, Tennessee, Florida, Mississippi, Kentucky, and Illinois) 421 days
Region V (Illinois, Ohio, Michigan, Indiana, Wisconsin, and Minnesota) 501 days
Region VI (Texas, Louisiana, Arkansas, Oklahoma, and Louisiana) 393 days Region VII (Missouri, Nebraska, Illinois, Iowa, and Kansas) 390 days
Region VIII (Montana, Colorado, Idaho, Wyoming, Minnesota, North Dakota, South Dakota, Iowa, and Utah) 402 days
Region IX (California, Nevada, Hawaii, Nevada, Utah, and Arizona) 290 days Region X (Oregon, Washington, and Alaska) 539 days

Like I said, you're in for a long and bumpy ride.

2. What can I expect at my SSDI hearing?

Make sure you understand the hearing procedures. The ALJ, your attorney (if you have hired one) and a vocational or medical expert, or both, will be present.

Be ready to answer questions from the judge. Questions you will be asked may include the following: name, date of birth and Social Security number, height, weight and living arrangements. The judge will also ask how you spend your day and what activities you do.

If you talk about how you love horseback riding, you work in your garden four hours per day, and you love to work out, expect the judge to decide you could do sedentary work for 8 hours per day.

If a vocational expert is present they may also list jobs they believe you can work based on your age, work history, physical condition and transferable work skills. If you have hired a lawyer they will provide medical evidence that you cannot perform any suggested jobs.

If the judge asks you if you think you could work any of the suggested jobs and you answer yes, expect the judge to deny your case.

Judges may issue a decision at the hearing but nothing is finalized until you have received written notification. Unfortunately, due to the back log for decisions, this could take up to 6 months.

How do you hurt your case? Show up late wearing flip-flops and short shorts, have no idea about the process, fail to hire a lawyer, and just for good measure, throw in a bad attitude.

3. When do I appeal my SSDI denial?

If you meet the nonmedical requirements for SSDI and you are sure you cannot return to work, you have 60 days from the date of the denial to file an appeal (the SSA will allow five days for delivery). In most states the first appeal is a reconsideration. Other states allow claimants to skip the reconsideration and immediately request a hearing.

If you wait to file after the 60 day deadline you will have to file a new application (some exceptions exist if you can prove you missed the date for a very good reason).

4. Do I need a lawyer to file an appeal?

Although some SSDI claimants have the fortitude to face the challenges of the SSDI appeal process without legal help, many do not. If you are very sick, you have no one else to help you, or you do not understand what you need to prove to win SSDI benefits, it may be time to talk to a disability lawyer.

Many claimants who filed SSDI applications on their own will decide to hire lawyers if they are denied. Consider also, it is generally better to file an appeal then to simply file a new application over and over again.

5. How far back will I be paid for SSDI?

To determine how far back you will be paid the SSA will review your Alleged Onset Date (AOD). Regardless of the AOD, however, the SSA is most concerned about the date you stopped working or performing substantial gainful activity (SGA). Your AOD cannot be before you stopped working at an SGA level. Another consideration is whether or not your medical records can prove your AOD. For example, even if you stopped working, if there is no evidence that you are disabled until months later, it may be tough to prove you were disabled at the time you stopped working.

For arguments sake, however, let's say that your AOD and the date you stopped working are the same. The SSA will not pay more than 12 months of retroactive benefits. There is also a five month waiting period for SSDI benefits.

With this in mind, a claimant would receive the maximum back pay allowed if their alleged onset date was 17 months prior to the initiation of the Social Security Disability Insurance (SSDI) claim (17 months less the 5 month SSDI waiting period allows for retroactive benefits for 12 months prior to the SSDI application date).

6. How is SSDI different than unemployment benefits?

The Social Security Disability Insurance program is a disability program which provides monthly cash payments to workers and their qualifying dependents who have a severe mental or physical health condition which is expected to last for at least 12 continuous months. Claimants must have worked and paid taxes, earning work credits, to qualify for SSDI.

Unemployment benefits are weekly cash payments offered to workers who claim they are able to work but cannot find a job. To collect unemployment benefits a worker must become unemployed through no fault of their own (layoff or termination which is not related to the employer's job performance), and they generally have to have been employed for a specific length of time.

7. How long does it take to file my SSDI application?

Completing your SSDI application will only take as long as it takes you to file the proper forms. Consider, however, that you will not qualify for SSDI benefits if your condition is not expected to last for at least 12 continuous months, if you are working or making too much money, or if you do not have enough work credits to be considered insured by the SSA.

8. How long will an SSDI appeal take with a lawyer?

Many SSDI applicants assume that having a disability lawyer will allow them to bypass the thousands of other disability applicants and somehow catapult their disability application to the front of the disability processing line. Uh, no.

Unfortunately, a disability lawyer will not be able to expedite your disability application by allowing you to cut in line. They may, however, give you a better chance of winning at every appeal step, thereby potentially saving you time and ultimately money.

9. What does a lawyer do for the money?

SSDI disability lawyers can do the following:

=File all appeal paperwork
=Prepare arguments for the disability hearing
=Challenge the job expert at the hearing if they argue you can perform different types of work
=Prepare a brief for the administrative law judge outlining the case
=Answer all of your questions related to your case
=Review your medical records and get more information if they feel that your current medical documentation is not sufficient to prove you cannot perform substantial gainful activity
=Send additional information to the administrative law judge prior to the hearing

More and more disability attorneys are also helping claimants complete their disability applications or have someone in their office who performs this task. If this is something you need help with you should contact several attorneys to find out if they provide this service.

10. How much will the disability lawyer be paid?

Disability attorneys charge a fee regulated by federal law, which is usually the lesser of 25% of disability back pay up to a maximum of $6,000. Costs can increase if your case goes to the Appeals Council or federal court, but generally you won't pay more than $6,000. Little or no money is required up-front, and you're only charged a fee if you win your case.

Some lawyers, however, may charge small fees for copying or requesting medical files. Talk to your lawyer and make sure you understand the fee agreement prior to hiring them.

And yes, almost everyone has back pay so you will end up paying them something if they win your case.

11. How many work credits will I need for SSDI benefits?

Workers can generally earn up to four work credits per year and will need 20-40 work credits over the course of their employment to be considered insured. The number of work credits needed to qualify for SSDI benefits will vary based on the age of the claimant at the time of their disability and may be lower for younger workers. Work credits cannot be bought, sold, or borrowed but must be earned by the worker.

Contact the SSA if you have questions about the number of work credits you need to qualify for SSDI benefits.

12. Is SSDI only for those with a permanent disability?

SSDI is offered to claimants who have a health condition which is so severe that they are expected to be out of work for at least 12 continuous months. If your condition will last at least 12 months you can apply for SSDI benefits, even if you do not expect to be permanently out of work.

13. What if my condition improves?

If you believe your condition has improved and you can return to work, you need to notify the SSA and let them know you are seeking employment. Do not start working without first notifying the SSA. If you do return to work and do not notify the SSA, you could end up owing them back pay for the benefits you received.

SSDI fraud is a crime. If you are no longer entitled to SSDI and you continue to claim benefits, not only does this take money from those who are legitimately disabled and need help, you could be charged with a crime.

14. Denied twice, can a lawyer help?

If you have been denied SSDI benefits two times a disability lawyer may be able to help, but this will depend on why you were denied. Many claimants do not qualify for SSDI benefits.

For example, if you have a short-term condition, if you do not have sufficient work credits, or if you are working and making too much money when you apply for SSDI it will not matter whether or not you have a lawyer, you will be denied SSDI.

15. Why won't a lawyer take my disability case?

Disability lawyers work on a contingency fee basis, and lawyers will not take your case if they do not think they can win. For example, if you do not meet the most basic requirements for SSDI- your condition will not last 12 continuous months, you do not have enough work credits for SSDI, your condition is not severe, or you are working too much- a lawyer will simply decline to help you.

16. Why was I denied SSDI?

Carefully review your denial letter. It should clearly state why you were denied. If the SSA states you do not have enough work credits for SSDI (and they did not miscalculate) then you may be able to get SSI, but you will never be approved for SSDI unless you go back to work and earn more credits.

What if the SSA says your condition is not severe enough or you can work another job? Assuming you meet all of the other nonmedical requirements, it may be possible for a disability lawyer to review your medical records and develop an argument, supported by great medical proof, that you cannot work another job and your condition is, in fact, severe.

17. How can I generate work credits for SSDI?

According to the SSA, the number of work credits needed for SSDI will vary based on your age you become disabled. For older workers this means you will generally need approximately 40 work credits. Twenty of your work credits, however, must have been earned in the last 10 years ending with the year you became disabled.

You can generally earn four work credits per year. The amount of earnings needed to generate a work credit varies and is periodically increased.

18. Can I borrow work credits from a spouse?

No, unfortunately, all work credits for SSDI must be earned through your own work and paying taxes. You cannot buy, steal, or borrow work credits from another person or from the Social Security Administration.

19. No work credits but I cannot work. What are my options?

If you do not have enough work credits for SSDI but working is out of the question then you can apply for Supplemental Security Income (SSI) benefits. SSI benefits are provided to the aged, disabled, or blind that are unable to work for at least 12 continuous months. Although you will not need work credits to qualify for SSI benefits, you will only qualify if you have very limited income and resources. Also, if you are married and your spouse has substantial earnings it is likely that you will not qualify for SSI benefits, regardless of whether or not you are severely disabled and you cannot work.

20. Can I file a reconsideration on my own?

Yes, you have 60 days to file the Reconsideration paperwork and submit it to the Social Security Administration (SSA). If you do not file the paperwork in time, under most conditions, you will have to file another SSDI disability application and start the process again. Consider as well that the back pay calculation will also restart and you will only get back pay back to the most recent application date, less the five month waiting period.

21. How do you file your own Reconsideration?

If you have received a medical denial you can appeal the decision online by going to the following link www.ssa.gov/disabilityssi/appeal.html You can also go to www.ssa.gov and type appeal my SSDI decision into the search box at the top of the screen. Additionally, medical decisions may also be appealed by completing the Request for Reconsideration, Form SSA-3441, Disability Report - Appeal, and Form SSA- 827, Authorization to Disclose Information to the Social Security Administration.

22. What is the difference between SSI and SSDI?

Social Security Disability Insurance (SSDI) is provided to disabled workers who have a severe health condition and who are unable to work for at least 12 continuous months. Unlike SSI benefits, an SSDI applicant must have worked and paid employment taxes into the SSA system to be considered "insured" for benefits.

Supplemental Security Income (SSI) is provided to the aged, blind, or disabled who are unable to work for at least 12 continuous months. SSI does not require applicants to have worked or paid taxes, but claimants must have very limited income and resources to qualify.

SSI payments are substantially lower than SSDI benefits. SSI claimants will also not qualify for Medicare, but will, in most states, be eligible for Medicaid.

23. Unemployment is gone. Should I apply for SSDI?

When you applied for unemployment benefits you were basically telling the federal government that you had the capability to work, in fact you were seeking employment, but you just had not been able to find a job.

If your unemployment has ended and you are considering filing for SSDI benefits the question you need to ask yourself is whether you cannot actually work or whether you simply cannot find a job.

You will not qualify for SSDI if the SSA believes there is work you could do given your age, work history, transferrable work skills and education level. If for instance you used to be a nurse and you know you can no longer do this work, the SSA may assume you could retrain for a sedentary job such as a medical data entry worker.

24. What do I need to know about SSDI before I apply?

Not everyone will win SSDI benefits.
It will be tough to win SSDI without great medical care.
You will not win SSDI without sufficient work credits.
Don't wait for the Social Security Administration to do all of the work.
Talk to a disability lawyer if you get denied.

25. I sent application to the SSA why have I not heard from them?

According to the Social Security Administration, there are more than 2 million disability

Past Relevant Work

As part of the Five Step Sequential Evaluation process the SSA will review whether a claimant is able to do past relevant work, which includes all work the claimant has performed within the last 15 years. If a claimant can perform past relevant work they will be denied SSDI benefits.

Physical Residual Functional Capacity

The physical residual functional capacity is the ability of a claimant to perform physical work functions. This capacity may be evaluated by a consultative examiner at a consultative examination. The CE will complete a residual functional capacity form (RFC) which details the claimant's ability to lift, carry, crouch, kneel, stoop, reach overhead, and perform fine motor functions.

Presumptive Filing Date

The presumptive filing date is the date a claimant notifies the SSA of their intention to file a disability application. After giving notification the claimant has six months from the date to submit and complete their SSDI application. This process is generally utilized if a claimant's date last insured (DLI) is near and the claimant wants to ensure they prior to this date.

Sequential Evaluation Process

The Sequential Evaluation Process is a five-step evaluation process utilized by the SSA to determine if a claimant is disabled and qualifies for benefits. The questions asked during this process include whether or not the claimant is working and making too much money, whether the claimant's condition is severe, whether the claimant's condition meets or exceeds a listing on the SSA Listing of Impairments, whether the claimant can work past relevant work, or whether the claimant can retrain for new work.

Social Security Administration (SSA)

The Social Security Administration was created when Franklin D. Roosevelt signed the Social Security Act of 1935. Currently, the SSA administers disability, retirement, and survivor benefits. Currently there are 1400 nationwide offices, including processing centers, field offices, hearing offices, and regional offices.

Social Security Disability Insurance (SSDI)

Social Security Disability Insurance (SSDI) offers wage replacement benefits to workers who are disabled, unable to work for at least 12 continuous months, and who have sufficient work credits to be considered insured by the SSA.

Substantial Gainful Activity

Substantial gainful activity (SGA) can be gainful work, which generates a certain amount of earning for a claimant each month, or substantial work, which means a claimant can work a specified number of hours, regardless of the income generated. Claimants who can perform substantial gainful activity are considered not disabled, regardless of the severity of their health condition.

For example, if you are a volunteer worker who works 40 hours per week the SSA is likely to deny your claim even though your work is not profitable. Their argument is that if you can do this many hours of volunteer work you have the ability to get a wage paying job.

Trial Work Period

The SSA encourages claimants to try to return to work. With this in mind, the SSA has created a program which allows a claimant to continue to receive SSDI disability benefits for a specified time period without jeopardizing their SSDI payments. Talk to the SSA if you want to return to work and you are receiving SSDI. If you work more than allows under the trial work program you will lose your benefits.

DO NOT GO BACK TO WORK WITHOUT FIRST TALKING TO THE SSA.

Work Credits

Work credits are earned by claimants as they work and pay employment taxes. All SSDI applicants must have a specified number of credits to qualify for SSDI. If you do not have enough work credits to be insured for SSDI, you will be denied. It does not matter if you cannot walk or you are in a coma. The SSA does not consider the severity of your condition if you are not insured.

applications submitted in any given year. This means there are millions of SSI and SSDI applications which must be reviewed and analyzed. Given the understaffing and the common inefficiency of the federal government, it's not surprising that it can take months to review a SSDI application.

26. Who will request my medical records?

Assuming your case meets the nonmedical requirements for SSDI and your case is sent to the DDS, they will request your medical records from all of the treating sources you have listed on your disability application. The SSA will not pull every single medical record but will request specific dates of treatment.

Getting medical records from doctors, however, can be the most time-consuming part of the disability process. Although electronic medical records transfers have been implemented for some treating sources, the process is not complete, and sometimes medical records have to be copied and sent to the SSA.

With this in mind, if you want to reduce the time it takes to be approved and you have recent and relevant medical information it is a good idea to give it to the SSA. Talk to the SSA representative about the best and most efficient way to provide them with your medical information.

27. Will I receive medical insurance if I qualify for SSDI benefits?

If you are approved for SSDI benefits you will get Medicare benefits within 24 months from your date of entitlement. Note: SSI claimants will not get Medicare benefits but will get Medicaid in most states.

28. Can I work part-time and get SSDI benefits?

It may be possible to work very part-time and qualify for SSDI benefits. Working too many hours, regardless of pay or profit, or making too much money, however, will eliminate your chance to receive benefits.

If you are receiving SSDI now and want to return to work the SSA does have programs which may allow you to attempt to work. This program is referred to as the Trial Work Period. Google Trial Work Period for SSDI and find out the specifics of the program.

Talk to the SSA before returning to work. If you work too much and do not notify them, you could owe them back payments or lose your SSDI benefits.

29. Can my wife and children get SSDI benefits?

Auxiliary benefits may be paid to the spouse or children of a disabled worker who is receiving SSDI benefits. To qualify, children must be under the age of 18, enrolled in full-time school, and not married. Spouses who are under the age of 62 will only qualify for auxiliary benefits if they are caring for a child under the age of 16, exceptions exist if the child is disabled.

Family members of workers receiving Supplemental Security Income (SSI) benefits are not eligible for auxiliary benefits.

30. SSA says my disability started after my date last insured (DLI) what does this mean?

SSDI is more like insurance than SSA retirement. What this means is that as you work you are paying premiums to ensure you are insured if you become disabled and unable to work. If you stop working for an extended period of time, at some point in the future, you will no longer be insured; this date is referred to as your date last insured or DLI.

You can call the SSA to find out your date last insured, but if you file for disability after your DLI date you will be denied. Your option, if this occurs, is to prove through medical evidence that your disability started prior to your date last insured.

Another option, if your DLI is approaching, is to talk to the SSA about establishing a protective filing date. This allows you to initiate the application and file before your DLI even if you are not able to complete the filing process.

31. What if I cannot afford medical care?

One of the most common issues for claimants is getting good medical care. This can be especially true for claimants who have been out of work and who do not have medical insurance. There is no good answer about how you can see a doctor without medical insurance. The best answer is to do the best you can.

Go to primary care clinics consistently until you build up a comprehensive medical file, or find a doctor who is willing to take cash payments for services. In some cases certain claimants may also qualify for Medicaid. As a last resort you may have to rely on county services and free clinics.

32. What if I go back to work before the medical decision and then inform the SSA after your claim has been approved?

If you return to work before the medical decision and then tell the Social Security Administration sometime after your claim has been approved the SSA will send the claim back to the DDS so they can modify the original decision to a denial. Unfortunately, if you received any SSDI payments these will be considered overpayments and will have to be repaid back to the SSA.

Glossary of Terms

Activities of Daily Living

Activities of daily living are all the activities individuals do each day:household chores, driving, shopping, fixing meals, socializing, paying bills, and personal hygiene and grooming. The assumption is that if a claimant cannot perform the basic activities of daily living they most likely cannot perform full-time, substantial work.

Information about a claimant's activities of daily living is collected on Form SSA- 3373 Functional Report or recorded by telephone on Form SSA-5002.

Administrative Law Judge

The Administrative Law Judge (ALJ) is employed by the Social Security Administration but works for the Office of Disability Adjudication and Review (ODAR). The U.S. is divided into regions and judges will preside over cases in specific areas.

All claimants who request a hearing will have their case reviewed in court by an Administrative Law Judge who will determine whether or not they are disabled. If the claimant disagrees with the judge's decision they may file another appeal to have their case reviewed by the Appeals Council.

Alleged Onset Date (AOD)

The alleged onset date is the date the claimant claims they were not able to perform substantial gainful activity due to their disability. The AOD may or may not be the same as the established onset date, which is the date the SSA states the claimant became disabled.

The EOD and the AOD may not be the same if the SSA cannot find medical evidence to support the claimant's AOD or the claimant performed work after their EOD.

Appeal

If a claimant's application is denied they may file an appeal, generally a reconsideration, within 60 days from the date of the denial letter. If their claim is denied again they may request a hearing. A final appeal may be made to the Appeals Council if a claimant does not like the judge's decision.

All other appeals after the Appeal Council appeal must be made outside of the SSA disability process through federal courts.

Auxiliary Benefits

Auxiliary benefits are benefits paid to the spouse or children of a disabled worker who is receiving SSDI benefits. To qualify, children must be under the age of 18, enrolled in full-time school, and not married. Spouses who are under the age of 62 will only qualify for auxiliary benefits if they are caring for a child under the age of 16, unless the child is disabled.

Family members of workers receiving Supplemental Security Income (SSI) benefits are not eligible for auxiliary benefits.

Award Letter

Claimants who are awarded SSDI benefits will be sent an award letter. This letter is sent via mail and contains information about a claimant's estimated date of their first payment and the amount they will receive.

Back Pay

Back pay is money paid to disability claimants because it has taken so long to process their disability claim. Back pay is calculated for SSDI based on the established onset date. SSDI applicants can only receive a maximum of 12 months back pay. Back pay is generally paid in one lump sum payment for SSDI recipients, but if you hired a disability lawyer their fee will be deducted from your back pay before the SSA sends it to you.

Blue Book

Blue Book is the informal name for the SSA Listing of Impairments, which apparently used to be contained in a blue book. Now, you can find the Listing of Impairments, which is a list of the most common conditions and their corresponding symptoms, online by googling SSA Listing of Impairments.

Claimants who have a condition on this list with the corresponding symptoms will be determined automatically disabled, assuming they have medical evidence to support their case and have met the nonmedical requirements of SSDI.

Close Period

Claimants who are unable to work for at least 12 continuous months may apply for SSDI benefits. If the claimant returns to work after 12 months but before they are awarded SSDI benefits, they may receive what are termed closed period benefits. These benefits are paid for the number of months the claimant was denied but no on-going disability is paid.

Compassionate Allowance

The Compassionate Allowance List is a list of the most severe conditions which the SSA agrees are disabling. Claimants who have a condition on this list will be allowed to have their SSDI application fast-tracked. The five-month waiting period still applies and claimants will still have to wait 24 months to receive Medicare (exceptions apply), but at least they avoid some of the hassle.

Consultative Examination

Claimants who apply for disability benefits but do not have sufficient medical evidence to prove their claim may be required to go to a consultative examination. This exam allows a doctor to perform a cursory review and notify the SSA of their findings. Most claimants report that these examinations do little to help them win benefits.

Date Last Insured (DLI)

Your date last insured is the last date you are covered under Social Security Disability Insurance. Let me explain. SSDI is more like car insurance and less like SSA retirement. Like car insurance you pay a certain amount each month so if you have a car accident you will receive compensation for medical bills and property damage. For SSDI, you pay employment taxes each month so you can be insured in case you become permanently disabled.

Also like car insurance, if you stop paying your premium, at some point in the future you are no longer insured. In this case, if you had a car accident the car insurance company would not pay for damages.

SSDI it works the same way. If you are working and paying taxes you are insured. If you stop working and stop paying taxes there is a point in time in the future will you will no longer be insured and will not be eligible for SSDI; that's your date last insured.

Denial Letter

Up to 70% of first time applicants will have their case denied. If your case is denied, the SSA will send you a denial letter. This letter will state the medical documentation the SSA used to make their disability determination, the reason the claim was denied, and the steps you can take to appeal the denial decision.

Disability Advocate

Disability advocates are individuals who specialize in helping disability claimants win disability benefits. Unlike disability lawyers who have a law degree, disability advocates do not have a legal juris doctorate but do have a bachelor's degree or equivalent qualifications and training and have passed a written test administered by the SSA which qualifies them to act as an advocate for claimants.

Disability Determination Services

Disability Determination Services include state agency and field offices which review disability applications after the SSA local field office has determined the claimant meets the nonmedical requirements for disability. DDS offices are funded by the federal government.

Disability Examiner

Disability examiners work at the Disability Determination Services offices and evaluate an SSDI claimant's application to determine if the claimant is disabled and qualifies for SSDI benefits.

Five Month Waiting Period

The SSA has instituted a five month waiting period to receive SSDI benefits. The five month waiting period starts on the established onset date.

Listing of Impairments

Also called the Blue Book, the Listing of Impairments is a list of common conditions and their corresponding symptoms that the SSA has determined are automatically disabling.

Medical Evidence

Medical evidence is all information gathered from a claimant's doctors. The SSA will review a claimant's most recent medical records to determine if they have a mental or physical health condition which is so severe it does not allow the claimant to work.

Medical evidence is the most important part of the disability decision making process. GET GOOD MEDICAL EVIDENCE.

Medical Expert

Medical experts may attend the SSDI hearing to provide medical testimony to the court concerning a claimant's mental or physical health condition(s).

Medicare

Medicare is health insurance provided by the federal government to individuals who are 65 years of older or who are under 65 years of age and receiving Social Security Disability Insurance. Medicare is not provided to SSDI claimants, however, until 24 months after their date of disability.

Nonmedical Requirements

Nonmedical requirements are those requirements which have nothing to do with a claimant's medical condition. For example, claimants who are working too many hours and making too much money or those who are not insured for SSDI will not qualify for SSDI because they do not

Additional Information

Social Security Administration Homepage
www.ssa.gov
(Make sure you are on their site. There are a lot of posers)

SSA Legal Information:

Social Security Act, The Code of Federal Regulations (CFR 20)
Social Security Rulings (SSR)
The Vocational Expert Handbook
https://ssa.gov/appeals/public_experts/Vocational_Experts_(VE)
_Handbook-508.pdf

Helpful Disability Sites:

www.disabilitycasereview.com
www.justipedia.com
www.disabilitybenefitshome.com
www.findlaw.com
www.disabilitysecrets.com/

Helpful Links:

Listing of Impairments
List of the most common health conditions and their symptoms.

Legal Disclaimer

This guide is not intended as legal advice. The author is not an attorney. The author is only providing this manual as a guide to those individuals who are floundering in the black-hell-hole of the Social Security Disability process and need a bit of practical advice.

Seriously, you must not rely on the information in this guide as an alternative to legal advice from your attorney or other professional legal services provider. If you have any specific questions about any legal matter you should consult your attorney or other professional legal service provider. You should never delay seeking legal advice, disregard legal advice, or commence or discontinue any legal action because of information in this guide.

This author is not an employee of the United States government or of the Social Security Administration. The views expressed in this work are solely the opinions of the Author and in no way represent the official views or policies of the SSA.

Furthermore, users should understand that the federal government periodically, and without provocation, updates disability laws, leading to more confusion for millions of disability applicants every year. Amazingly, the government does all of this without ever getting advice from this author.

About the Author

Beth Losure currently lives in Dallas, Texas, with her husband and three children. She is a contributing writer for LeadRival, the leading provider of pay per action advertising for legal services, and Justipedia, a legal encyclopedia. She has also spent time over the last several years as a case worker for a disability attorney's office, and a forum moderator for a disability website. In her spare time she teaches English as a Second Language to immigrants from all over the world.

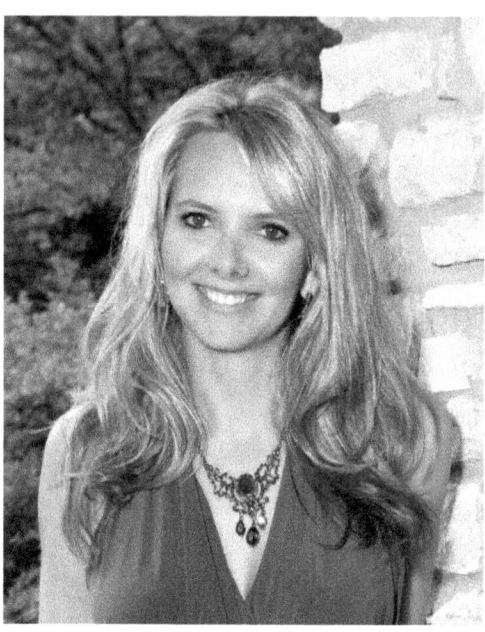

www.ingramcontent.com/pod-product-compliance
Lightning Source LLC
Chambersburg PA
CBHW081251180526
45170CB00007B/2381